Praise for *Physician of Souls*

Jeanne Stevenson-Moessner has refl
interface of healing and faith. Now
to a winsome expression. She sees t
faith and medicine is entirely permeable, and she easily crosses
the line between the two. This book will be both a welcome
instruction and a moving motivation for those who seek to find
well-being in the wise, generative practice of faith.

—Walter Brueggemann, William Marcellus McPheeters
Professor Emeritus, Columbia Theological Seminary

This book is a masterful revisioning of the common concepts
around ministry and healing. With fierceness and authority,
Stevenson-Moessner weaves narrative vignettes with theology,
medical research, and church history to highlight the uniqueness
of holistic, multivalent care. She artfully critiques assumptions
about religion, sin, suffering, and healing through the lens of
culture and gender to invite readers to another level of understanding about the minister's role in dealing with the sick, the
broken, and the marginalized.

—Bishop Teresa E. Snorton, DMin, ACPE, BCC (retired),
ecumenical and program development officer,
The Christian Methodist Episcopal Church

With immense knowledge and experience, Rev. Dr. Jeanne
Stevenson-Moessner brings us this important work on "physicians of the soul," which describes a vital ministerial role for our
present time. We need more "soul healers" since the concept of
health is more wide-ranging and broader than many of us imagine. Ministers and practitioners of medicine have much to learn
from each other, and we can all listen better to those who suffer.

—David Markham, MD, cardiologist, Atlanta, Georgia

Jeanne Stevenson-Moessner summons her deep pastoral experience and a wealth of personal insights to bring the late-fourth-century preacher John Chrysostom's vision of "a physician of souls" to life as a compelling model for multireligious healing ministries in the present-day world. Her reflections on real-life examples at the intersection of religion and medicine today are especially thought-provoking, and compellingly call for a more integrated approach to health and healing.

—Margaret M. Mitchell, Shailer Mathews Distinguished Service Professor of New Testament and Early Christian Literature, University of Chicago

Jeanne Stevenson-Moessner has captured the art and science of medicine in the words of a faithful and dedicated theologian and pastoral care giver. In these pages you will find what it means to be totally committed to a ministry far beyond anything you have ever experienced. She drives home the power of what can be, when everyone is on the same page when it comes to healthcare.

—Rev. Dr. Charles R. Millikan, Dr. Ronny W. and Ruth Ann Barner Centennial Chair in Spiritual Care, and vice president for Spiritual Care and Values Integration, Houston Methodist Hospital

Jeanne Stevenson-Moessner "breathes new life" into Chrysostom's concept of "physician of the soul." This book is a must-read for clinical pastoral education students and chaplains who strive to make meaning of their call in a clinical environment.

—Rev. Willacin "Precious" Gholston, BCC, MDiv, MPP, Certified Educator in the Association for Clinical Pastoral Education

Jeanne Stevenson-Moessner mines the wisdom of John Chrysostom for contemporary spiritual care, teaching us what it means to be a "physician of souls." This pastoral theology of healing elevates the chaplain's role in healing the fullness of mind-body-souls, while also emphasizing pastoral accountability through a "credo of caregiving," analogous to the Hippocratic oath. The author's moving stories illustrate soul-full ministry as medicine.

—Mary Clark Moschella, Roger J. Squire Professor of Pastoral Care and Counseling, Yale University School of Divinity

In this evocative book, Stevenson-Moessner envisions a theology of healing that embraces a model that bridges spiritual care and medicine in service to care of the entire person. She invites pastors and chaplains to reclaim their rightful place as those who tend to the dis-eases of the spirit and to recognize that spiritual maladies, often shaped by those in power, require us to act boldly in renaming and reclaiming on behalf of the marginalized. Stevenson-Moessner introduces a fundamental frame for guiding caregivers in the crucial task of soul care, from which we can all benefit.

—Rev. M. Jan Holton, PhD, associate professor of the practice of pastoral theology and care, Duke Divinity School

With insight born from deep faith, lived experience, and scholarship, Jeanne Stevenson-Moessner explores the two worlds of medicine and ministry, and the languages inherent in both endeavors. She names the shared missions and priorities, while simultaneously probing tensions and illuminating new understandings of "body, mind, and spirit" for all who are called to vocations in the healing professions, whatever they may be.

—Mary Lynn Dell, MD, MTS, ThM, DMin, academic physician and Episcopal priest

PHYSICIAN
of SOULS

PHYSICIAN
of SOULS

MINISTRY AS MEDICINE

Jeanne Stevenson-Moessner

FORTRESS PRESS
Minneapolis

PHYSICIAN OF SOULS
Ministry as Medicine

Illustrations:
Extending Arms of Christ Mural by Bruce Hayes used by permission
of Houston Methodist Hospital.
The Dollhouse, photograph by Gwen Gross Miller. Used by permission
of Jeanne Stevenson-Moessner.
The Trinity, Petru Botezatu, photograph by Gwen Gross Miller. Used by
permission of Jeanne Stevenson-Moessner.
The Seven Deadly Sins, Jean Stevenson Moessner
© Jeanne Stevenson-Moessner. Used by permission.

Library of Congress Cataloging-in-Publication Data

Names: Stevenson-Moessner, Jeanne, author.
Title: Physician of souls : ministry as medicine / Jeanne
  Stevenson-Moessner.
Description: Minneapolis : Fortress Press, [2024] | Includes
  bibliographical references and index.
Identifiers: LCCN 2023048539 (print) | LCCN 2023048540 (ebook) | ISBN
  9781506496627 (print) | ISBN 9781506496634 (ebook)
Subjects: LCSH: Health--Religious aspects. | Medicine--Religious aspects. |
  Religion and medicine. | Spirituality.
Classification: LCC BT732 .S725 2024 (print) | LCC BT732 (ebook) | DDC
  261.5/61--dc23/eng/20240117
LC record available at https://lccn.loc.gov/2023048539
LC ebook record available at https://lccn.loc.gov/2023048540

Cover design: Kristin Miller
Cover art: Spring, Edvard Munch, 1889, oil on canvas

Print ISBN: 978-1-5064-9662-7
eBook ISBN: 978-1-5064-9663-4

To Linda and Dale Wlochal of Dubuque, Iowa,
Who stepped in as our Dubuque family,
Who made certain our children were never latch-key,
Without whom I would not have produced
my early books,
Without whom we would have missed laughter,
UNO, good food.
When the Dubuque airport was closed in winter
weather,
Dale drove me all-night to my presentation in
Atlanta.
Dale, thank you for your service to our country.
I count my blessings and dedicate this book to you
both.
Jeanne Stevenson-Moessner, May 24, 2023

Contents

Contents

Acknowledgments

Writing an acknowledgments page is like counting my blessings. I am repeatedly grateful to Fortress Press for their support and for their renewed commitment to pastoral theology. Bethany Dickerson has been a diligent editor. Lindsey Johnson Edwards, my research assistant, has enriched each chapter with her own experience and knowledge of healthcare. Lisa Eaton and Sarah McNamee have diligently seen this work into production.

I am thankful to work at an institution that promotes research. President R. Gerald Turner and Provost Elizabeth G. Loboa of Southern Methodist University have taken many measures to promote faculty research, writing, and publications. I am indebted to Perkins School of Theology for a fall release time in 2022 and a Scholarly Outreach Grant. Thank you to Jane Elder for her expertise with materials in Bridwell Library. I could not have made such progress without the condo in Dubuque, Iowa, which was provided by Dr. Jim Jerrard and Mary Lynn Neuhaus during my release time. It was my hiding and writing space.

The Native American Conference, "Healing with Dignity: Spiritual and Pastoral Care in Native America," was made possible by a generous grant from The Association of Theological Schools and the Henry Luce Foundation. Colleagues Dr. Michelle Oberwise Lacock, Rev. Carol Lakota Eastin, Pamela Goolsby, Carolyn Douglas, and I worked conscientiously to create a safe and hospitable space for forty-five members of Native

American tribes who gathered several days at Perkins School of Theology. I was honored to listen in and learn.

Colleagues at Perkins School of Theology have taught me much. In regards to this book, Dr. Jaime Clark-Soles has given me tutorials in the current research on psychedelic-assisted therapy. Students enrich my understanding; I am indebted to Richard Pokoo and Sylvanus Chapman for their interviews. There are others who contributed to this book, but have chosen to remain anonymous. Thank you for your trust and your narratives.

For those who have encouraged me specifically these last months in the writing of this book, I thank Rev. Amy Fowler, Rev. Paul and Donna Moessner, Dr. Evon Flesberg, Rev. Dr. Susan Sharpe, Judy Haskins, Dr. Martha Robbins, Rev. Amos and Sarah Disasa, Sara Staley, Marie Sommerfelt, Dr. Bonnie Sue Lewis, Anne and Robert Sayle, Rev. Fran Shelton, Rev. Mary Stewart Hall, Janace Grant, Leigh Frazier, Lyann Korbyn and Jessica Tamlyn, Rev. LeNoir Culbertson, The Moessners, Rev. Beth McCaw, and Jane Lange. Thank you, Kelley Coutee, for your guidance and insights. My two lively granddaughters, Vida Fae and RhyLee Jean Davison, bring light and life into my life.

For the Class of 1966 at St. Mary's Episcopal School and former students who have faithfully kept in touch, I am blessed. Thank you to Ashley Moore Remmers and Angie Keesee for their trip to Dallas and to Lucy Walt Wepfer for her remembrances. For the continuing ties with St. Mary's Episcopal School in Memphis and for the faith of that school in me, I am humbled. For the chance to teach at Houston Methodist Hospital, for the collegiality of the staff, for the chance to work with Rev. Dr. Charles Millikan and Rev. Stacy Auld, I am a better person.

My family is more than a blessing. My husband Dr. David Moessner and my daughter Jean Moessner are a source of encouragement, centering, and love. My son David Moessner, who is at home with God, is present to me in ways not of this earth.

At Madison Heights Methodist Church in Memphis, as a child I sang this song: "Count your many blessings, name them one by one." I am off key sometimes, but I am still singing.

Jeanne Stevenson-Moessner,
September 2023

Author's note

The sermons on Matthew which contain references to "physician of souls" are all taken from *St. John Chrysostom Homilies on the Gospel of St.Matthew (I-XLV)* edited by Paul A. Boer, Sr. (Edmond, Oklahoma: Veritatis Splendor Publications, 2012) and excerpted from *A Select Library of the Nicene and Post-Nicene Fathers of the Christian Church*, edited by Philip Schaff, LL.D. (Buffalo: The Christian Literature Company, 1886), vol.7. These homilies or sermons by Paul Boer are in English.

The Greek text that is often used in this book regarding "physician of souls" is taken from the work of Fridericus Field AA.M. in his collection Johannis Chrysostemi, Archiepiscopi Constantinopolitani, Scribebam Cantabrigiae, vol. I, Homilies 1–45, Cambridge, England, 1839, at the expense of the editor.) Below is the last section of Chrysostom's Homily 29 on Matthew 9: 1,2. Found on page 414 in Field's text.

Και τα Χριστω δε ηνίκα προσήεσαν οι μαθηταί αξιούντες πυρ καταβηναι εκ του ουρανού, σφόδρα επετίμησεν αυτοις λέγων: 16 « ουκ οίδατε ποίου πνεύματός έστε υμείς." Και ενταύθα δε ουκ είπεν, ώ μιαροί και γόητες υμείς ώ βά σκανοι και της των ανθρώπων σωτηρίας έχθροί αλλά, τί

ενθυμείσθε πονηρά εν ταις καρδίαις υμών;" Δει τοίνυν μετ 'Β επιεικείας εξαίρειν το νόσημα. "Ο γαρ φόβω γενόμενος ανθρωπίνω βελτίων, ταχέως επανήξει προς την πονηρίαν πάλιν. Διά τούτο και τα ζιζάνια αφεθηναι εκέλευσε, διδούς προθεσμίαν μετανοίας.

Πολλοί γουν

αυτων μετενόησαν, και γεγόνασι σπουδαίοι, πρότερον όντες φαυλοι, οίον ο Παύλος, ο τελώνης, ο ληστής και γαρ ζιζάνια όντες

ουτοι σιτος γεγόνασιν ώριμος. Ἐπί μεν γαρ των σπερ μάτων τουτο αμήχανον επί δε της προαιρέσεως, ραδιόν τε και εύκολον "ου γαρ φύσεως όροις αύτη δέδεται, αλλ' ελευθερία προαιρέσεως τετίμηται." Όταν τοίνυν ίδης έχ θρόν της αληθείας, θεράπευσον, επιμέλησαι, προς αρετήν

επανάγαγε, βίον επιδεικνύμενος άριστον, 17 λόγον και παρε C χόμενος ακατάγνωστον, προστασίας και κηδεμονίαν παρέ

χων, πάντα τρόπον κινων διορθώσεως, τους αρίστους των ιατρων μιμούμενος. Ουδε γαρ εκείνοι καθ 'ένα τρόπον θερα πεύουσι μόνον, αλλ' όταν ίδωσιν ούκ είκον το έλκος τω προ τέρω φαρμάκω, προστιθέασιν έτερον, και μετ 'εκείνο πάλιν άλλο και νυν μεν τέμνουσι, νύν δε επιδεσμούσι. Και συ τοίνυν ψυχών ιατρος γενόμενος, πάντα κίνει θεραπείας τρόπος κατά τους του Χριστού νόμους, ίνα και της σαυτον σωτηρίας

και της ετέρων ωφελείας λάβης μισθον, εις δόξαν θεου πάντα D ποιών, και ταύτη και αυτός δοξαζόμενος.

18 • Τους δοξάζοντας γάρ με δοξάσω, φησί και οι εξουθενουντές με εξουθενω θήσονται." Πάντα

τοίνυν εις δόξαν αυτού πράττωμεν, ίνα της μακαρίας εκείνης και επιτύχωμεν λήξεως' ης γένοιτο πάντας ημάς επιτυχείν, χάριτι και φιλανθρωπία του κυρίου ημών" Ιησού Χριστού , και η δόξα και το κράτος εις τους αιώνας των αιώνων. Αμήν.

Prologue

Igrew up in a medical family. I knew that doctors were highly respected. I was born a girl so I did not consider becoming a doctor. I was not encouraged to be a physician, rather the wife of a professional. I later chose to be a chaplain. In the hospital during my clinical pastoral education training, I walked with my head slightly bent, intimidated by the men in white coats. Two decades later, I also passed women in their white coats, who briskly walked along the same corridors. I made way for them and was always deferential. Theirs was the critical work in the hospital.

One day, as adjunct professor at a Protestant seminary, I attended a fall faculty retreat far away from the seminary. I left the retreat early to return home to my small children. Before I got home, the seminary receptionist called me: a seminary student and her husband were in a serious car accident. The seminary student was in the critical care unit in a coma.

I was the only faculty member near the hospital.

I got there and waited three hours while the nurses and doctors tried to stabilize the seminary student. I visited with the parents and was prepared, by them, for what I would see in the Intensive Care Unit (ICU). The parents left to get some rest, and I stood alone in the hallway outside the ICU, waiting and feeling helpless— as medical personnel rushed in and out of the ICU. After all, it was up to the medical staff to stabilize and save her. Theirs was the critical work in the hospital.

When the nurse told me I could enter, I did my deep breathing and faced the machines and the tubes and the fragile boundary between life and death. I prayed a pastoral prayer close to the student's ear and mentioned by name those who loved her and were praying for her. I touched the student's pale arm to give her a sense of human warmth, and I made the sign of the cross with holy oil, invoking the power of the Trinity. Following these sacred ministrations, I, as chaplain, left and returned to the same hallway where I had felt helpless and passive.

However, upon returning, I felt fierce. Fierceness is waiting when you cannot alter the situation. Fierceness is going into nursing homes and facing senile dementia and Alzheimer's when some of the medical profession cannot. Fierceness is staring into the face of suffering. Fierceness has nothing to do with passivity, and everything to do with fervent conviction. After this difficult visit, I never again felt inferior to physicians of the body. I hold my head high and proudly wear my badges whether chaplain or minister.

Even today, many years later, I contemplate the mystery of the healing of this student. Was it entirely medical intervention, or the prayers of those who believe in a God who heals, or a combination of both? I do not know, but of this, I am certain: I am a physician of the soul, and I hold my head high.[1]

NOTE

1   This encounter is described in detail in my chapter "Incarnational Theology: Restructuring Developmental Theory," in *In Her Own Time*, ed. Jeanne Stevenson-Moessner (Minneapolis: Fortress Press, 2000), 9.

ONE

Spirituality and Healing

It was always a special day when Mr. Colter drove in from Germantown, Tennessee, with a pick-up truck full of vegetables, meat, and watermelons from his farm. Mr. Colter was a regular patient of my father. Dad let him pay for his medical care with produce from his farm. Back in the 1950s, I never thought to ask whether this patient was underinsured or uninsured. He was treated with great respect and dignity, and that is what I saw and knew.

Today, the phrase *house calls* is not used very much as far as I can tell. For my two brothers and me, the phrase was as easily understandable as the words *medical office*. Dad often made house calls for his elderly patients. If they were dying alone, he would sit by their bedside, sometimes through the night.

The hardest memory for me is the night when the phone rang after we had all gone to bed. My brothers, younger than me, had been asleep for a while. I pretended to be asleep, but I was reading under the covers with my flashlight and heard the conversation between my father and a suicidal patient. The patient was thanking my father for all the care given to him. He thanked dad for all he had done as his doctor. Then he said, he could no longer go on. He had a gun, and he had placed the life insurance papers close beside him for his wife to find. Dad said all the right things that are taught in suicide prevention training. Dad asked him to put the gun away, that he was coming right over. Suicide prevention training also teaches that sometimes one fails to prevent what another has determined to do. Dad failed. He lost a longtime patient that night. It is a painful memory for me. This loss for him was soul-wrenching.

My father was a doctor of internal medicine. He was not a psychiatrist, and in the 1950s and early 1960s, I doubt suicide prevention training was as prevalent as today. My father had learned both the science and the *art* of medicine, the aim of accomplishing a holistic *good*.[1] His respect and care for his patients and his belief in their dignity and worth undergirded the curative methods and aims of biomedical science. His respect and care was reciprocated in many ways by his patients – even in honoring him with the last phone call.

As a physician of internal medicine, he sat at his oak desk and listened to patients describe the context of their lives. His patients sat in a green armchair and told of their aches and pains, their grief and frustrations. Once in his office I noticed something unusual. When I commented on all the *unopened* medical journals on his desk, he told me: "I spend a lot of time listening." Health care, for him, was multivalent. He prescribed medicine, performed clinical procedures, took X-rays, and gave physicals. When his patients were dealing with grief issues, he prescribed a sad movie and told them to have a good cry. It was not uncommon for him to sit by the bedside of elderly patients when they were dying, especially if they had no family. For him, medicine was a ministry. This term, medicine as ministry, has been developed by pediatrician Margaret E. Mohrmann.[2] Dr. Mohrmann, Professor Emerita of Biomedical Ethics, UVA's School of Medicine and Department of Religion, explains that "anyone who teaches clinical medicine will have observed that hospitalized patients in medical centers often love the green third-year medical students assigned to them, and look upon them as their primary doctors during their hospital stay."[3] One of the reasons for this, she believes, is that the nervous medical student, not remembering all of the appropriate questions for particular complaints, often ends up just listening to the patient's flow of words. Describing these medical students, Dr. Mohrmann concludes that "they do not know enough to direct the story into the structured lines that they are taught to use. Consequently, their patients feel that they have finally been heard by someone."[4]

When my father retired in 1990, he gave me his oak desk and the green chair in which his patients sat. I, a minister, theologian, and pastoral counselor, now sit at his oak desk in my office at Perkins School of Theology and spend a lot of time listening. From that same green chair, I hear at times stories of joy, accounts of healing, and realizations of calling; I also hear at times existential pain, spiritual scarring, and internal anguish. I have become a physician of the soul, and as such, I offer ministry as medicine.

This phrase, "physician of souls," originated with John Chrysostom, a patristic writer in the fourth century CE.[5] John Chrysostom was concerned with diseases of the soul and advocated for the use of every means of cure. I have chosen the term "physician of the soul" because it is a connective term. It is a phrase that links those of us who primarily tend to soul-destroying emotions, spiritual distress, or existential agony to those who primarily tend the physical bodies of the suffering or to those who treat those facing distresses of the mind (psyche). I envision that if teamwork strengthens among various types of caregivers, from physicians of the body to physicians of the soul, then we will probe deeper into the art, science, and mystery of healing. I am using the term "dis-eases of the soul" to highlight not only the pathology of a soul infected with deceit, bitterness, hatred, regret and other contaminations of the health of a soul, but to offer a contrast to a soul imbued with honesty, magnanimity, love, peace, and other conditions for spiritual wellbeing. The health or illness of the soul will always impact the fitness of the body and mind.

We begin this journey with listening. A physician of the soul listens to the patient's flow of words. Physicians of the body can do so as well. The late Nelle Morton, theologian, feminist, and activist, offered the concept of "hearing a person into speech."[6] This notion reflects a God who listens intimately and intensely, hearing even the sound of the silent tear fall. Another theologian, feminist Riet Bons-Storm from Holland, reminds us to hear the silence before the speaking.[7] If we do this as physicians of the soul, we shall hear stories, the silences before the stories, and the new images that surface in the telling of the stories. As the medical model becomes more fast-paced, regulated, and standardized, this shift creates a need for more teamwork among chaplains, doctors, nurses, and pastors. We will need to listen more intentionally to the context of patients' lives. This listening is not a mimicking or parroting of what the patient says. It is a listening with the ear of God for the subscripts, for the narrative unfinished, for the story not even born.

A physician at Erlanger Hospital models this type of listening. Betty Terry was on the janitorial staff at the hospital when she asked Dr. Clif Cleaveland, MD, MACP, to be her doctor. Her many years of sweeping, mopping, and emptying waste cans had taken a toll on her fatigued joints, but she never complained. Her concern was about a malignancy on her face. It was a nodule, the beginning of an abnormal growth or neoplasm, that would eventually take her life. The surgery cut into the mandible and the neck. Radiation failed to keep the tumor in check.

Dr. Cleaveland entered a sacred space with Betty Terry. He began to grasp the fallacy of a physician taking the patient's history.[8] "This story, if honored with time and privacy, defines an immediate illness or problem not as some isolated calamity but as part of a continuity of experience. This history speaks to the dream and fears, regrets and joys of a unique person."[9] Cleaveland further defines this sacred space between doctor and patient and the mystique of medicine. He writes,"Now I realize the incompleteness of medical education based solely upon science. Medicine is not simply a branch of chemistry or the biological sciences. Clinicians especially live among stories: those of their patients and their colleagues and those that seek expression within their own souls."[10] This is the listening my father, Nelle Morton, and Margaret Mohrmann, MD, were conveying. The sacred space between patient and doctor contain stories "toward uncertain destinations. Some of these voyages are over, some are still underway. These journeys have taught me to be more aware of my own. The sacred space is where our journeys coincide."[11]

HEALING AND RELIGION

In ancient times, the healer and the priest were the same person.[12] Giving advice on treating illnesses was one role and privilege of the priest, the learned and holy man. Today, we experience a bifurcation of the healer and the priest/pastor/imam. Yet, the sacred space where our journeys coincide is the very place where we can collaborate and participate in the healing of body-mind-soul. This is hallowed ground where medicine is ministry, and ministry is medicine.

History affords numerous examples of the healer and the religious leader being one and the same. In 1536, the three ships commanded by Jacques Cartier, French explorer, were frozen in the St. Lawrence River near Montreal. A terrible scourge had broken out among the confined sailors. Twenty-five percent of the sailors had already died by the time a First Nations chief, Domagaia, became involved. Domagaia ordered his men to boil limbs of a spruce tree. This was made into a tea which was administered to the dying men. The men recovered and lived. Two hundred years later, it was discovered that vitamin C was the cure for scurvy, the disease from which many of the sailors died. Vitamin C was found in many plants including the spruce. First Nations people knew of the healing resources of many indigenous plants, some used today for medicinal compounds.[13] In the Hebrew Bible, Jehovah-Rapha was the God who healed.[14] Prophets of this God were gifted in healing. One example is that of Elisha, a prophet who healed Naaman of leprosy.[15] In the New Testament, Christ emerges as the One who came to heal. John Chrysostom stated it in these terms: "For He hath come as a Physician, not as a Judge."[16] One of the Buddhas, Bhaishajyaguru, is the Medicine Buddha. In the temple of Jogyesa in Seoul, South Korea, he is depicted as holding a gallipot, a small jar containing medicine or ointment. It is claimed by followers that both spiritual and physical ailments can be cured. In Greek mythology, Asclepius was the god of healing and his daughter Hygeia, was the goddess of health. In ancient Egypt, the goddess Sekmet had multiple roles, but she was recognized as a remarkable healer. She was the patron deity of physicians and healers.

In many cultures, the religious leader (or god) was the healer. My goal in underscoring this connection is to make further advances in recapturing this connection. The connection between spirituality or religion and healing accrued renewed interest when researchers at Harvard Medical School, Deaconess Hospital, quantitatively linked spirituality and healing and brought forward new evidence in the mind-body-spirit connection. I became interested in this connection when I attended an early conference in Boston in 1996, The Spirituality and Healing conference, under the leadership of cardiologist Dr. Herbert Benson.[17] This conference spurred my interest in contributing to an holistic approach to the interconnection of the mind (*psyche*), the body (*soma*), and the soul/spirit (*die Seele/pneuma/ruah*). My particular focus is to highlight and explore the religious leader's role in the healing phenomenon of mind-body-soul. I am using the word "soul" as the core of our being where the Holy, the Higher Power, the Wholly Other, or the Holy Spirit links with our spirit through creation and through experience. In our medically advanced and clinically specialized culture, the role of physicians of the body and physicians of the mind in the phenomenon of healing are much more clearly and scientifically defined. I begin with a complicated case that will raise issues about medicine, ministry, and miracles and the roles of healers: physicians of the body, mind, and soul.

MEDICINE, MINISTRY, MIRACLE

Mrs. Mattingly's Miracle documents the healing of the widowed sister of Washington's mayor. This "miracle" became a polarizing event, not only in Washington, but in the Roman Catholic Church.[18] In March of 1824, a woman encased in bed sores lay limp on her bed; her medical diagnosis was end-stage-breast cancer. Her breathing was shallow with rattles; the tumor on her left breast was huge and prevented her from moving her arm. Her illness had lasted seven years. As her friends and doctors gathered around her, the smell of vomit and diarrhea was in the air. The doctors knew she was in the end stage of life. And yet, her family was hopeful that "if God can touch the human psyche, God can touch the body as well, and both psychological and physical healing [can] become a religious possibility."[19]

However, a group of her friends, along with some Catholic priests, had written Prince Alexander Hohenlohe, a famed and charismatic healer and priest from Baden-Wuerttemberg in southern Germany, to cure her. Although Hohenlohe's main ministry of healing occurred in Europe, by the second and third decades of the nineteenth century, seventeen healings in America had been attributed to him. He was gaining an "international" reputation. Under Hohenlohe's instructions, a *novena* or a set of prayers would be offered at sunrise by members of Ann Carberry Mattingly's parish of St. Patrick's in Washington, DC. On the tenth day, if members were faithful in the *nouvena*, he would offer his prayer for her healing at Mass in Bamberg, Germany. This would be another one of Prince Hohenlohe's long-distance healings. Simultaneously, the three parish priests of St. Patrick's would offer her the Eucharist in Washington, in her room.

On March 10, 1824, Rev. Stephen Dubuisson appeared with a small ciborium, which contained the Holy Eucharist. Ann Mattingly's tumor was so inflamed that she could not reach the Host. The priest put it on her parched tongue after a severe coughing spell. The Host stuck in her mouth for five to six minutes as she struggled to swallow.

Sacred silence engulfed the room, crowded with friends and family. As some were still kneeling at the bedside and praying, she arose from the bed praising God. She walked to the table that had served as an altar for The Eucharist and bent her knee. The lump on her breast was gone, her bed sores and ulcers were no more, and her pulse was normal. Her brother, Thomas Carbery, mayor of Washington, DC exclaimed, "All this complicated machinery of the human system, so much deranged and out of order, beyond the reach of medicine and medical skill, was, in the twinkling of an eye, restored to the most regular and healthful action."[20]

Ann Mattingly lived thirty-one more years. Her "miracle cure" was heavily documented, as was the custom in the Catholic Church. Researcher Nancy Lusignan Schultz has methodically analyzed this miracle from several perspectives and from extensive research. For example, from a *political perspective*, this miracle gains prominence because Ann's brother was mayor of Washington, DC at the time. Ann's brother compared her healing to that of Lazarus in the New Testament. From a *religious perspective*, in 1824, Catholicism was strong and respected in the area around Washington, DC. The Catholic community was open to miraculous healings and was careful to interview and document. From a *gender perspective*, women were considered the weaker sex and used by God in their weakness to confound the world. From a *medical perspective* in the early nineteenth century, Nancy Lusignan Schultz noted, "As was typical with nineteenth-century female invalids, her male physicians partially attributed her maladies to gynecological problems."[21]

On the day of "Ann's Miracle," Prince Hohenlohe did not hold a healing mass; he was on vacation. Secondly, although he was in the process of being examined for sainthood in the Catholic Church, his name was withdrawn amid accusations of promiscuity, indebtedness, and lasciviousness.[22] Nevertheless, eyewitness accounts heralded his healings, both distance and in person, throughout Europe. He had many adherents and many opponents. Still, Ann Mattingly was healed.

We are all mortal, and we shall die. We survive illnesses and viruses that are reversible, that is, by regaining wellness or health. However, sooner or later, we face "'the sickness unto death' whether it comes through accident or through virus or through bacteria or simply through the fact that we wear down, wear out, and die."[23] In Ann Mattingly's case, she was facing "sickness unto death" with stage four cancer. This is the reason her healing was designated as a miracle. It was perceived as a healing from a single source. In Mattingly's case, the singular cause of healing was prayer.

In the twenty-first century, this issue of healing comes with different spiritual worldviews of the interface of religion and modern medicine. Morton Kelsey offers a classic study of historic shifts in an understanding of healing miracles.[24] There was a healing ministry in the early Christian church. However, Protestant theology became greatly influenced by Martin Luther and John Calvin, both of whom rejected miracles.[25] According to Kelsey, other theological influencers such as Karl Barth did not deny nor affirm the contemporary healing ministry.[26] It is rare for a mainline theological school today to offer a course in healing. The gifts of prayer, preaching, administration, mercy and hospitality, for instance, are presented through "bona fide" seminary/divinity school courses. Healing is too sensitive and radical a subject. In his historical review of healing, Kelsey noted that "the academic side of Christianity has shown little interest in the Christian healing ministry."[27] People will have varying approaches to the interconnection of spirituality and healing. The dialectic between faith and reason may be activated. "The story of the Mattingly miracle is threaded through with questions of the porous border that separates doubt and belief."[28]

There have been a number of studies that have proven quantitatively that prayer is efficacious. Earlier in this chapter, I referred to the work from Harvard's Deaconess Hospital under the guidance of Dr. Herbert Benson, MD.[29] This cardiologist and surgeon stressed the science and power of belief. As mentioned at the beginning of this chapter, Benson and associates were able to prove quantitatively that patients who engaged in a "relaxation response" such as prayer or yoga before surgery did better during surgery and postoperatively. The patients left the hospital earlier, and this drew the attention of CEOs and boards of hospital systems. In 1988, Dr. R. C. Byrd produced data from 393 coronary care patients in a double-blind protocol that indicated intercessory prayer had a beneficial effect on patients in the Coronary Care Unit, specifically less ventilatory assistance, less antibiotics, less diuretics.[30]

In the case of Ann Mattingly, all medical interventions and devices in 1824 were exhausted as she entered into stage four breast cancer. The sole cause of her healing was attributed to prayer of the faithful. However, in the studies of Dr. Herbert Benson, prayer was prelude and part of the healing. The outcome indicated that prayer was efficacious during surgery and postoperatively, but prayer was not the sole cause of healing. In Dr. Byrd's study of patients in coronary care, prayer resulted in a greater state of wellbeing.[31] My term *multivalent healing* is meant to capture the use of various types of medicinal, therapeutic, pharmaceutical, surgical, communal, and prayer support that all could play a role in healing. When a patient recovers, it could be a combination of two or more of these approaches. I am using the adjective "multivalent" as a way to honor these different interpretations, applications, meanings, and causes.

In earlier times, the healer and the priest were often the same person. Giving advice on treating illnesses was one role and privilege of the priest, the learned and holy man. Today, we experience a bifurcation of the healer and the priest/pastor/imam. Yet, the sacred space where our journeys coincide is the very place where we can collaborate and participate in the healing of body-mind-soul. This is hallowed ground where medicine is ministry, and ministry is medicine.

MEDICINE AND MINISTRY JOIN IN CARE FOR THE DYING

In his acclaimed work on failed treatment of dying children and resulting medical care at the end-stage of a child's life, pediatric psychologist David J. Bearison uses numerous clinical cases/clinical narratives to illustrate the painfully challenging task of providing care to the child, the family, and the caregivers themselves.[32] In these clinical write-ups, the nonfamilial caregivers are the medical personnel including doctors, nurses, the occasional social worker, and the priest.

In one of the scenarios involving a mother and her critically ill young son, a social worker served as a go-between for the medical staff and the bewildered mother. "The social worker was unbelievable . . . She was the one person that the mom could talk to, and the mom knew that she understood her and she would be able to tell us [medical staff] exactly what she [mom] wanted."[33] Especially in a teaching hospital with numerous teams making rounds and with intense medical discussions going on at the bedside, family members can be overwhelmed.

In a different scenario, a nurse is comforted by the priest at the child's funeral: "The funeral was helpful to me because the priest echoed the words I had been telling the family all along, which confirmed that I had done the right thing for them in helping them . . . I heard back from the priest, what I had told them, which was helpful because this was a mind-blower, the whole thing. The priest said to me, 'You took very good care of this family and they have the utmost respect for you.'"[34] Other medical professionals expressed a desire to have someone to talk to after the loss of a child. One doctor referred to the defenses that have to go up so a doctor can be strong.[35] Other doctors hesitate to overload colleagues with their personal debriefing of a loss. Residents don't feel prepared to deal with the dying child or the family. The role plays in medical school are not adequate.[36] One medical staff gets to the heart of the problem: "My real issue is that I still don't know what's the right way to say farewell to the families."[37]

The psychological and emotional overloading and the feelings of inadequacy and incompetency, and others that follow, express tender and sensitive places where chaplains and religious leaders can help. After all, medical staff are trained to cure patients. They are not trained in most medical schools for the final farewell— the death of a patient. As examples will indicate in the next sections, medical professionals can feel helpless at the bedside of a dying patient when there is nothing more that they can do. They have spent years training to heal. On the other hand, chaplains spend years training to face their own mortality and that of those for whom they care. This complementarity in training could make a profound partnership.

BEING IMMORTAL

"Medical professionals concentrate on repair of health, not sustenance of the soul" writes Atul Gawande, MD, in *Being Mortal: Medicine and What Matters in the End.* "It [medicine] has been an experiment in social engineering, putting our fates in the hands of people valued more for their technical prowess than for their understanding of human needs."[38] Then he advocates for a more accepting, compassionate, appropriate, humane understanding and approach—by the part of the medical profession—to mortality and death.

In 1969, my college roommate had to be transported in the middle of an ordinary, weekday night to Vanderbilt Hospital's Emergency Room. Eventually, she was transferred to the Intensive Care Unit. I do not remember how anyone in that ICU would have known that I was the chaplain of a sorority on campus. Perhaps my roommate told them. All I remember definitively is that a nurse came to the waiting area and asked me to help a family who had just lost their father/husband. Of course, I was stunned by this request. I had no formal training to do what was being asked. Yet, I moved forward into a more private waiting room off the ICU where a traumatized family huddled together.

At that time, the ICU at Vanderbilt Hospital in Nashville was constructed in a circular formation with the nurses' stations in the middle. This way every patient could be seen from that nurses' station unless a curtain was drawn over the patient's cubicle. As I sat in the middle of the family made up of children of various ages, some of whom were young adults, we could actually see their father's cubicle where he lay—dead—on his cot. His wife, their mother, wept at his bedside. He had been involved in a car accident and injured beyond repair.

To this day, I cannot recall anything I said to that family. They knew I was a "chaplain." I sat in the middle of them, somehow feeling part of their pain, although I had not yet experienced the great tragedy of death in my life. I may have let a tear fall. If they had asked me to hold their hand, I am sure I complied. Mainly, I sat in the middle of them, confronting with them this boundary between mortality and immortality that their father had crossed as we watched. They were Catholic; I am Protestant. In a sacred space like death, the little cubicles we build around our faith groups dissolve in the face of a greater reality. I recall that I was asked to pray when the mother returned to us. I stayed in their suffering for some time until they were ready to go.

The equivalents of chaplains and priests in other world religions are usually the ones trained to stand on this boundary between mortality and immortality. There are different understandings of immortality depending on the religion or philosophy. It generally means an existence of the soul and often the body after the death of the body—death in medical terms.

As a Protestant minister and chaplain, I am now trained to go to the frontlines of suffering. We chaplains, ministers, priests, rabbis, and other clerics do not sit on the sidelines of suffering. We do not do the work of the medical profession or that of hospice and palliative care. Rather, we are physicians of the soul. As Atul Gawande states honestly: "But scientific advances have turned the processes of aging and dying into medical experiences, matters to be managed by health care professionals. And we in the medical world have proved alarmingly unprepared for it."[39] Historiographer Mary Dunn writes from her experience with cancer: "There is an alienation that becomes the patient newly diagnosed with disease. It is modern medicine's particular achievement, however, to sever the patient slowly and steadily from the specificity of her own story (witness the plastic wrist bands, the generic and ill-fitting gowns, the standardized questionnaires about developmental milestones, pain and quality of life)."[40] She further adds that her book, *Where Paralytics Walk and the Blind See: Stories of Sickness at the Juncture of Worlds,* is an exercise in meaning-making for those suffering from illness, disease, accident, ageing or embodied difference. As she faces sickness and her daughter Aggie lives with disability, it is a clear possibility to fall into a narrative authored by the medical authorities. However, as Mary Dunn and her daughter control their own narratives and make meanings of their lives, they also become authors of their lived experience: "The measure of our lived experiences with sickness and disability could not and cannot be captured by the meanings made within the therapeutic treatment rooms of the modern hospital."[41] The restitution narrative is dominant in modern hospitals where the restitution is the "cure." For many patients like Dunn who are seeking to make their own meaning of their bodily illnesses or physical limitations, they choose to compose their own meaning-making narrative. This time of meaning-making is often the place where a chaplain, minister, imam, priest, or pastor can sit (figuratively or actually) and listen in to the script. "Physicians of the soul" can also—when appropriate and desired—offer guideposts along the way.

Now, we as physicians of the soul are being increasingly prepared to accompany the aging and dying, the young who are dying. We are also being prepared for the curing and healing of *dis-eases of the soul.* This is our work. We sit and move in very sacred spaces. We are involved in a realm much larger than ourselves. I believe this is why I was unafraid in that waiting room at Vanderbilt Hospital.

MEDICINE AS MINISTRY, MINISTRY AS MEDICINE

Dr. Margaret Mohrmann used the term medicine as ministry. The reverse application is also true. Ministry can supplement medicine. Dr. Aoife Abbey, a physician and registrar in intensive care in Britain, has written honestly and humanly of the complex feelings of doctors, nurses, and other medical personnel in her bestselling work, *Seven Signs of Life: Unforgettable Stories from an Intensive Care Doctor.*[42] Dr. Abbey was newly certified as a physician. Her ninety-year old patient was nearing death and was deeply frightened. She was frail and failing with pneumonia. Her constant plea, "'Please don't let me die,'" communicated her anguish. She was alone in a side room in an elderly care ward. Dr. Abbey tried to soothe her; she made sure her patient was given medications to make her comfortable. Still Gloria was gripping her in desperation: "I felt in that moment more powerless than I had ever expectedly to feel."[43] She called the consultant on the ward and asked if the family was aware of the situation. Together they phoned the family and met with them. The family suggested a chaplain would bring Gloria comfort: "It seemed like such a straight-forward and obvious answer. Why did

I not think of it myself? Confronted by her fear, I had panicked because I had no medical solutions."[44]

Two chaplains came and took turns being with Gloria. Dr. Abbey passed by her room many times and always saw a chaplain seated close, with "their hands folded on their lap in that peaceful way they do. Gloria died that night . . . I believe the chaplains gave her what she needed—that which I couldn't give her—and I don't think she died frightened."[45] This is the fierce, faithful, and formidable work that we as physicians of the soul are both trained and called to do. We are prepared to sit in the sacred spaces, especially as one whose body has failed is making the transition to the realm of spirit. This is ministry as medicine.

Three years later, Dr. Abbey arrived at the hospital early and noticed one of her patients, ninety-four years of age, in the throes of death. She sat, took his hand, looked into his eyes, called his name, and said comforting words. "He was quiet then and his two hands wrapped themselves around mine: bones drenched in skin."[46] He died 20 minutes later—but he did not die alone. This is medicine as ministry.

There are times when the medical staff themselves need comfort as they deal with fear, grief, distraction, anger, disgust as well as joy and hope. We as chaplains and other forms of physicians of the soul are also trained and called to be there for them in these moments. I end this chapter with the longing and expectation that not only can the multivalent ways of healing be acknowledged but the collaboration among those tending the body, the mind, and/or the soul will enhance our mutual goals of beneficial caregiving.

I recall the story a young seminarian told me of one of his first nights on call in a Dallas hospital. He was a chaplain-in-training. He was called to a room filled with family members crowded around a man who had just died. The deceased had been husband, father, grandfather, uncle, brother to those wailing, screaming, crying in the shock and agony of this sudden loss. The seminarian knew immediately that it was a warm, demonstrative, closely knit family who deeply loved this man. The noise was so loud that the seminarian stood in the corner of the small room with his badge on his jacket: CHAPLAIN. After a long while, the raw emotions settled into quiet crying and sighs. He stayed—in the corner—until every family member had the time they wanted. He went back to the chaplains' offices, feeling he had failed. The next afternoon, he was stopped in the hallway by a family member whom he remembered from the night before. Before he could say one word, she clasped him tightly and with profound gratitude, thanked him for all he had done for the family. She said: "We could not have made it without you." She squeezed again, then left. Amazed, he told me later: "I never even said one word."

We chaplains and pastors are trained in grief work and techniques appropriate for a situation like this. Many times, we know that what is needed is a presence that does not flinch from pain, does not dominate the situation, does not flinch in the face of death, chaos, or the cacophony of grief. We know that we represent faith in the face of death; we can be present with others in great pain, and we can be partners with medical staff as we offer ministry as medicine.

THE CASE OF ANNE O'CONNELL: PART 1

Reflect on this chapter with its focus on spirituality and healing, the bifurcation of religion and medicine, and the partnership or lack thereof of the players in this true case.

In March 1976, Anne O'Connell[47] of Wisconsin noticed a pain in her right lower leg, just below the knee. She was employed at Mercy Hospital as a licensed practical nurse on a medical floor. The hospital was understaffed and quite busy. Anne O'Connell kept working hard until the third week of March. The pain in her leg grew and it hurt to be working at such a fast pace. The assistant head nurse approached and told her to go to the emergency room. Anne declined saying: "I need to take care of my patients." Later, she was approached again and told that other nurses would tend her patients. When she entered the emergency room, a well-respected surgeon saw her and ordered X-rays. Next, she was seen by an orthopedic surgeon who informed her of her test results. The diagnosis was osteogenic sarcoma of the right fibula. This was a rare form of bone cancer. Anne said: "Not much was known about this cancer or how to treat it. My parents were told that I was at death's door. My cancer was grade four. I was encouraged to be seen at Mayo Clinic in Rochester, MN. I was stunned." She was twenty-three years old.

She visited an abbey which was ten minutes from her home. Her family frequently visited this abbey, and her mother had grown up on a farm nearby. Her grandfather and the monks helped each other tend their fields. She and her cousins would walk over together to the abbey to see Father Pius who ran the gift shop. Father Pius had come to the abbey from Ireland when he was nineteen years old. Father Pius was lighthearted and kind; he was an inspiration to her. Her mother explained to Father Pius her situation, and he asked to see her before she left for Mayo Clinic. "Father Pius met and prayed with my mom and me." She was anointed with holy oil and given a sacred relic. Friends, relatives, and parish priests were all called for prayers. She was remembered at weekly masses. She felt the strength of these prayers as she left for Mayo Clinic the last week of March 1976. She and her parents sat in waiting rooms for five days as tests were run. Anne noticed that people from all over the world surrounded her with that same look of being scared and stunned. After five days of tests, she had an appointment with her orthopedic surgeon, Dr. F. H. Sims. He had been on a team of surgeons that performed the surgery for Senator Edward M. "Ted" Kennedy Sr.'s son, Edward Moore Kennedy, Jr. on November 17, 1973. Young Edward had been twelve years old when osteosarcoma, a form of bone cancer, was diagnosed in his right leg, below the knee. The leg was surgically amputated above the right knee.

NOTES

1 My father's clinic emulated Robert Sokolowski's description of the art of medicine. On this term, Sokolowski writes, "An art is the ability to accomplish a good. An appreciation of the good to be done is programmed into the art, programmed not as one more step in its procedures but as saturating every step from beginning to end. Medicine as technique is what is left over when the medical art is drained of its sense of the good . . . But what is the good of the medical art? It is the health of an individual or community." For a fuller articulation of the art of medicine, see Robert Sokolowski, "The Art and Science of Medicine," in *Christian Faith and Human Understanding: Studies on the Eucharist, Trinity, and Human Person* (Washington, DC: Catholic University of America Press, 2006), 241.

2 Margaret E. Mohrmann, *Medicine as Ministry: Reflections on Suffering, Ethics, and Hope* (Cleveland: Pilgrim Press, 1995).

3 Mohrmann, *Medicine as Ministry*, 66–67.

4 Mohrmann, *Medicine as Ministry*, 66–67.

5 John Chrysostom, "Homily XXIX," in *Homilies on the Gospel of St. Matthew* (I-XLV), ed. Paul A. Boer, Sr. (Scotts Valley, CA: CreateSpace Publishing, 2012), 362.

6   Nelle Morton, *The Journey is Home* (Boston: Beacon Books, 1985), 202.

7   Riet Bons-Storm, *The Incredible Woman: Listening to Women's Silences in Pastoral Care and Counseling* (Nashville: Abingdon Press, 1996).

8   Clif Cleaveland, MD, *Sacred Space: Stories from a Life in Medicine* (Philadelphia: American College of Physicians, 1998), 207–10.

9   Cleaveland, *Sacred Space*, 208.

10 Cleaveland, *Sacred Space*, 26.

11 Cleaveland, *Sacred Space*, 210.

12 Matthews, Dale, MD "Plenary Address for the Spirituality and Healing Conference" (speech, Boston, 1996).

13 Porter Shimer, *Healing Secrets of the Native Americans: Herbs, Remedies, and Practices that Restore the Body, Mind, and Spirit* (New York: Tess Press, 1999), 44–45.

14 See example of Sarah's infertility in Gen 18:11–14; Gen 21:1–2.

15 II Kings 5:1–27.

16 John Chrysostom, "Homily III," in *Homilies on the Gospel of St. Matthew* (I-XLV), ed. Paul A. Boer, Sr. (Scotts Valley, CA: CreateSpace Publishing, 2012), 62.

17 Benson and his team were able to prove quantitatively that a form of spirituality, a relaxation response such as prayer or yoga, was efficacious in positive surgical results and faster post-operative recovery. Chaplains, ministers, and religious leaders were criticized for their lack of published scientific studies with quantitative analysis of their effectiveness. Fortunately, recent studies have documented effectiveness (See *The Faith Factor, Volume Two: An Annotated Bibliography of Systematic Reviews and Clinical Research on Spiritual Subjects* by David B. Larson, MD, M.S.P.H.) (National Institute for Healthcare Research, Presented to the John Templeton Foundation, December 1993).

18 Nancy Lusignan Schultz, *Mrs. Mattingly's Miracle: The Prince, the Widow, and the Cure That Shocked the City* (New Haven: Yale University Press, 2011).

19 Morton Kelsey, *Healing and Christianity: A Classic Study* (Minneapolis: Augsburg, 1995), 25.

20 William Matthews, *A Collection of Affidavits and Certificates, Relative to the Wonderful Cure of Ann Mattingly, Which Took Place in the City of Washington, D.C., on the Tenth of March, 1824* (Washington, DC: Georgetown University Library, Special Collections, 1824), 9.

21 Lusignan Schultz, *Mrs. Mattingly's Miracle*, 168.

22 Lusignan Schultz, *Mrs. Mattingly's Miracle*, 221.

23 Marjorie Hewitt Suchocki, *In God's Presence: Theological Reflections on Prayer* (St. Louis: Chalice Press, 1996), 58.

24 Kelsey, *Healing and Christianity*.

25 Kelsey, *Healing and Christianity*, 17.

26 Kelsey, *Healing and Christianity*, 18.

27 Kelsey, *Healing and Christianity*, 199.

28 Lusignan Schultz, *Mrs. Mattingly's Miracle*, 226.

29 Herbert Benson with Marg Stark, *Timeless Healing: The Power of Biology and Belief* (New York: Simon and Schuster, 1996).

30 Randolph C. Byrd, "Positive Therapeutic Effects of Intercessory Prayer in a Coronary Care Unit Population," *Southern Medical Journal*, 7 (1988): 826-29, Doi: 10.1097/00007611-198807000-00005.

31 There were four subsequent studies that were interpreted as disproving the Byrd and Benson studies into the efficacy of prayer.

32 David J. Bearison, *When Treatment Fails: How Medicine Cares for Dying Children* (New York: Oxford University Press, 2006).

33 Bearison, *When Treatment Fails*, 180.

34 Bearison, *When Treatment Fails*, 199.

35 Bearison, *When Treatment Fails*, 201.

36 Bearison, *When Treatment Fails*, 216–17.

37 Bearison, *When Treatment Fails*, 209.

38 Atul Gawande, MD, *Being Mortal: Medicine and What Matters in the End* (New York: Henry Holt and Co., 2014), 128.

39 Gawande, MD, *Being Mortal*, 6.

40 Mary Dunn, *Where Paralytics Walk and the Blind See: Stories of Sickness at the Juncture of Worlds* (Princeton: Princeton University Press, 2022), 25.

41 Dunn, *Where Paralytics Walk and the Blind See*, 151.

42 Aoife Abbey, *Seven Signs of Life: Unforgettable Stories from an Intensive Care Doctor* (New York, Arcade Publishing, 2019).

43 Abbey, *Seven Signs of Life*, 47.

44 Abbey, *Seven Signs of Life*, 47.

45 Abbey, *Seven Signs of Life*, 48.

46 Abbey, *Seven Signs of Life*, 74.

47 The name Anne O'Connell is a pseudonym suggested by the interviewee. I have also changed the name of the state in which she lives. Otherwise, the names of the priests, all physicians whether at Mercy or Mayo, and all spiritual retreat centers are actual and accurate.

TWO

John Chrysostom's Enigmatic Imagery

> Bestowing attention and tender care, by trying every means of amendment, in imitation of the best physicians, for neither do they cure in one manner only, but when they see the wound not yield to the first remedy, they add another, and after that again another; and now they use the knife, and now bind up. And do thou accordingly, having become a physician of souls.
>
> —John Chrysostom, "Homily XXIX"
> on Matthew 9:1–2

Several of John Chrysostom's images of healing are enigmatic when applied to religious professionals. Chrysostom offers the following for religious professionals: Cutting with the Knife, Imitating Physicians, Using Every Means of Cure (or Amendment), and Binding the Wounds.

What does Chrysostom mean for those in ministry, chaplaincy, and pastoral counseling when he urges us to cut as a surgeon? Most of us have been trained in reflective listening, empathic support, mechanisms of transference and counter-transference. We tend to create a safe space for disclosure, especially for those suffering from a trauma. We probe with gentleness, create an environment where no one is violated, and cultivate a nonjudgmental approach. Does "cutting like surgeons" translate into confrontative patient/church member/client care? What does that look like and how can it heal? Furthermore, for those of us in therapeutic, counseling, ministerial or chaplaincy relationships, Chrysostom's medical images are puzzling if not mysterious. How do we imitate physicians? How inclusive is "using every means of cure?" Without EMT, paramedic, or medical training, how do we "bind the wounds?" Before putting credibility into these analogies, it is important to know the nature and social location of the man who spoke them.

JOHN CHRYSOSTOM

John Chrysostom (ca.349–407) was a controversial, Christian bishop of Constantinople who left a concept that has not been given the attention it deserves in the field of pastoral theology, practical theology, ecclesiastical and ministerial studies. This concept is the ministerial description "physician of souls."[1] John Chrysostom was well-educated, and he was trained by the rhetorician Libanius. Chrysostom not only wrote countless influential sermons, but his deliverance of them was so eloquent and persuasive that he was called "goldenmouthed." His sermons and commentaries on the gospel of Matthew have given us the concept of ministers as physicians of the soul.

Chrysostom had many followers as a bishop, but he also acquired enemies. He "was frequently at odds with the monastic community due to his intense reform efforts."[2] For example, he disagreed with *subintroductae*, or spiritual marriage in which men and women celibates live together.[3] Chrysostom also regarded the city or *polis* such as Constantinople as the site for Christian ethics, formation, identity, and orthodoxy.[4] This understanding reflected his intense reform efforts. It was the power structure of the polis he hoped to reform. He preached that anything superfluous to one's basic needs should be given away to the needy. He was concerned about the poor of the city and advocated almsgiving to them as an antidote to the evil of mammon. He preached against the vast wealth of some citizens and suggested they take the poor into their homes. In short, he hoped to create an ideal city like the primitive church in the New Testament, a city of God. Chrysostom faced various forms of opposition, most notably from an enemy, Theophilus, who arranged for Chrysostom to be kidnapped at night, put on a ship against his will, and taken into exile. All of this occurred amidst theological debates such as the doctrine of the Trinity, ecclesiastical and political power plays, and Chrysostom's attempts to reform Constantinople. In his reformation tactics, it is said that "he was to degrade potent sites of imperial self-aggrandizement, such as the hippodrome, monuments, and statues."[5] Thus, Chrysostom's resistance to political and ecclesiastical abuse of power and authority did not put him in favor with the government. The moral stands that he made were based on his exegesis of Genesis, the Psalms, the Gospel of Matthew, the Gospel of John, and the Acts of the Apostles. Because of his theological and ethical stakes in the ground, Chrysostom was exiled twice, and he did not return from the second exile.

In the midst of this contentious and contagious context, Chrysostom was not deterred from his concerns for his flock. Chrysostom was concerned with *dis-eases of the soul* and advocated the use of every means of cure.

This patristic Greek and Christian concept, physician of souls, is not only currently relevant to the wounds of society, but to the pain of individuals as well.[6]

There are clues for religious leaders and theologians in their response to pain, illness, moral injury, soul-wounding, and crisis, using every means of amendment.

CHRYSOSTOM'S HOMILIES ON MATTHEW

In exploring the theological and biblical context from which Chrysostom developed the term—physician of souls—it is crucial to turn to his homilies or sermons on the book of Matthew. Chrysostom made it clear that Christ came as a physician, not a judge.[7] Referring to King Herod's anger at the news of the wise men or Magi, an anger that resulted in the slaughter of innocent children, Chrysostom speaks of Herod's soul: "For when a soul is insensible and incurable, it yields to none of the medicines given by God."[8] Chrysostom refers to Christ as the skillful Physician of Souls and encourages Christians to act in this manner. Chrysostom writes,

> Accordingly, when thou seest an enemy of the truth, wait on him, take care of him, lead him back into virtue, by showing forth an excellent life, by applying "speech that cannot be condemned." By bestowing attention and tender care, by trying every means of amendment, in imitation of the best physicians.[9]

Chrysostom has been regarded as a moral philosopher or an ethicist as well as a theologian. Using a proliferation of examples in his sermons of the Gospel of Matthew, he advocates the pursuit of virtue. Chrysostom rebukes his male audience for frequenting swimming pools in which naked harlots swim and preen themselves by swimming lengths of the pool.[10]

> But thou, having the fountain of blood, the awful cup, goest thy way into the fountain of the devil, to see a harlot swim, and to suffer shipwreck of the soul. For that water is a sea of lasciviousness, not drowning bodies, but working shipwreck of souls. And whereas she swims with naked body, thou beholding, art sunk into the deep of lasciviousness. For such is the devil's net; it sinks, not them that go down into the water itself, but them that sit above.[11]

He admonishes against watching women naked on a stage performing acts of adultery and intercourse as entertainment. According to Chrysostom, pornography puts to shame the common nature of woman. How does a man—after these evenings of watching such acts on a stage or after viewing women swimming naked—approach his wife upon returning home? He declares the wife more virtuous; therefore, she should be the authority in the home! And this is the remedy: she should instruct the husband! Because Christ's genealogy and birth are the focus of this Matthean homily, Chrysostom juxtaposes the harlot on the stage with the Virgin and Christ in the manger: "And seeing Christ lying in the manger, thou leavest Him, that thou mayest see women on the stage."[12]

By cutting deeper into the soul, Chrysostom might free the lascivious man "from the venom of them that intoxicate you."[13] By making the metaphorical knife sharper, he can cut deeper and eliminate that which is putrefied to become purified.[14] There are medicines or antidotes given by God if a soul is receptive. To be receptive, a soul must leave the theater of the devil or the evil machinations of Herod and like the wise men (Magi), turn to honor, adore, and follow the Son of God. The pursuit of virtue regards mammon as a pursuit of the wealth of power accumulated by any means. Chrysostom uses Herod as an example of being yoked to this dis-ease. Herod's monopoly of power was threatened by a little child for whom the Magi searched. Herod is dis-eased by the cancer of anger. He directs his anger to the most vulnerable: children under the age of two. This becomes the slaughter of the innocents in Bethlehem.

The dis-eases of the soul as listed in the Homilies on the Epistle to the Romans included ungodliness, unrighteousness, vile affections, reprobation, and deceit. The last dis-ease—deceit—is likened to the poison of asps under one's lips. This is why some dis-eases necessitated cutting with a knife: to remove the venom, the poison, the sepsis. The deadlier the infection, the sharper the knife to extrapolate the dis-ease.

The physician not only "plucks the dart" from the wound but also remedies are applied. God has come in Christ as the physician. He is the Redeemer of souls. He came to heal not to judge. He healed bodies in acts acclaimed as miracles while on this earth. Chrysostom proposed that Christ performed the healing miracles, primarily bodily healings, first so that Christ might be entitled to credit or credibility.

CUTTING WITH THE KNIFE

"For this cause I have made my language the stronger, that by cutting deeper I might free you from the venom of them that intoxicate you: that I might bring you back to pure health of soul; which God grant that we may all enjoy by all means."[15]

How do we envision "cutting with the knife" today as we, physicians of the soul, encounter spiritual toxins, contagion, sepsis, and malignity? Cutting with the knife means the extraction of something toxic, dis-eased, death-inducing. Cutting with a knife could be ameliorating defenses such as denial, for example, through confrontation in counseling. Other defenses include distortion, projection, dissociation, repression, reaction formation, displacement, intellectualization. Cutting with a knife could be the elimination of a toxic situation. Cutting with a knife could also be a means to assist the delivery or birth of some newness of life. It does not involve a literal knife that cuts into skin and draws blood. It is usually the professional use of skilled words. Here are two examples that may help clarify this concept.

I first observed "cutting with the knife" at Charter Peachford Hospital in Atlanta in the addictive disease unit to which I was assigned as a clinical pastoral education intern. In 1988, the nurses, therapists, social workers, and doctors were very blunt with patients in the addictive disease unit. In group therapy, the staff would cut through patients' defenses, denials, and excuses as with a sharp sword. They were extremely confrontative when met with falsehoods, lack of accountability, and passing the blame. As chaplain intern, I asked one therapist privately why this approach was healthy. She startled me with the recidivism rate, which was 70 percent. That means "more than 70 percent of people struggling with alcohol abuse will relapse at some point."[16] The therapist ended with this, and I paraphrase: "We are hard on them because we know their lives are at stake. We are confrontative so that more will make it."[17]

On the other hand, there can be gentle cutting in removing something festering[18]. In the movie, *The Kindness of Strangers,* a nurse in a hospital runs a support group centered around forgiveness. She is gentle, humble, soft-spoken, but focused and dedicated. All members of this group are desperately lacking in forgiveness toward someone or something. It is not at all clear that any members really see the importance of the centering issue in the support group: forgiveness. The members seem adept at externalizing all blame. Still, the nurse carries on in her gentle way although she carries a small scalpel, metaphorically speaking. After some time, she doubts her effectiveness and tells her superior that she will disband the group. Horrified, the superior puts her hand to her mouth and says there is a long waiting list for this group. There has been so much psychological healing reported, and word has gotten out! By the denouement of the movie, we as viewers see members of this support group dramatically offer "the kindness of strangers." It was the gradual, gentle work of a small scalpel—weekly cleaning the wound of festering unforgiveness.

There are times when physicians of the soul must utilize confrontation, as do physicians of the body and mind. Gordon Hilsman gives a plethora of examples from his work as a seasoned professional chaplain in using his authority to confront with empathy. For example, he has confronted medical care teams about the terminology "withdrawing life support" from a patient. This idea of withholding or taking away a lifeline can cause distress to family members who live with guilt for years. Hilsman offers a better, kinder term: allow them "a natural death."[19]

PHYSICIAN OF SOULS

As mentioned earlier, pastoral healers in the twenty-first century are often viewed as inferior in stature to medical healers, doctors of the mind and the body. We are not given the same authority in the clinical arena of health and wellness. Yet Chrysostom prescribed "applying the word without accusation, bestowing attention with authority and standing with the authority of a physician, a protector, one who shows care."[20] Religious professionals such as chaplains are known for taking a subsidiary position to medical personnel, especially in a hospital setting. Our salaries in comparison to medical professionals reveal our "market value." In her essay on "Medicine and the Market: The Misenchantment of Modernity," Lindsey Johnson Edwards presents a convincing case that the "role of the supernatural in medicine has been reduced to a mere coping mechanism for those who remain religious or spiritual".[21] The elevation of the scientific and the quantifiable on the seesaw of market value lowers the net worth of the spiritual, non-quantifiable, and qualitative analysis. The healthcare industry values quantitative data. The industry downgrades qualitative studies and data which is what ministers and chaplains provide. Yet, on another scale of value, when we religious professionals enter a hospital room, filled with machines, tubes, and pumps, we come with oil of anointing, we represent the faith tradition of the patient, we represent those in communities praying for the patient. We often stand at the boundary of life and death. Those religious professionals in the Christian tradition enter as an emissary of Christ the healer.

Pastoral authority manifests itself in many shapes and configurations. Pastoral authority is the exercise of wisdom that is accrued from two or more of the following: from formal pastoral training, from endorsement by a religious body, from the covenant or promise made at ordination to serve others and use gifts such as teaching and preaching; from the Holy Spirit. Every denomination or faith tradition has its own process of recognizing pastoral authority. In my denomination, The Presbyterian Church USA (PCUSA), there is a four-fold process to validate pastoral authority:

> Articulation of a clear inner sense that God is calling the person to an office of ministry requiring ordination; testing of that inner call by the church itself. In practice, this had included an examination not only of the person's knowledge and gifts, but also their way of life. Election to office by a particular community of God's people, ordinarily a congregation. Admission to the office (ordination) in the context of public worship, through prayer, with the laying on of hands.[22]

There are annual assessments each year after ordination. Pastoral authority is not about control, rather it is a commitment to serve and care for others, particularly the underserved in our society. In the two personal examples that follow, I was prompted to serve by what I believe, in retrospect, was the motivation of the Holy Spirit. The first scenario required that I use my pastoral authority to delegate, to take charge in overseeing, and to remain a non-anxious presence in the midst of a crisis. In the second scenario, I reached out for help from professionals through the Red Cross. This is a move we learn in pastoral training: to ask for help when we need it. I became the coordinator of a massive support response, and I was a counselor in the aftermath of what unfolded.

First scenario: While I was teaching a seminary course at The University of Dubuque Theological Seminary on the second floor, a student had an apparent heart attack at the end of a break. He rose and stumbled toward the hallway where he collapsed. With the sacred adrenalin that fuels pastoral authority, I rushed down the aisle of the class delegating responsibilities. I asked the one nurse in the class to call 911 and follow me to the hallway where she tended to the unconscious student. I asked another student who knew the student well to call his wife. I asked four students to go to the ground floor and each stand by an outside door to direct the responders to the one elevator. I asked another four other students to go to the door of each classroom on that second floor and keep all students inside. This was an old building, with narrow hallways, steep steps, sharp turns. It was a large class so I asked most to stay seated and pray. There was silence in that room. Those students may have thought they were playing the bit parts, but I wonder, in retrospect, how huge their role may have been. The emergency services did not waste a minute getting to us. They stabilized the student and took him quickly to Finley Hospital in Dubuque. He survived. I am not much of a delegator by nature, but on that day I stood "with the authority of a physician, a protector, one who shows care."

Second scenario 2: There are times when we physicians of souls speak with an authority that is not of our own. I was raised in Memphis, lived in Nashville while at Vanderbilt, moved back to Memphis to teach, went to Princeton for a degree, then to Europe for eight years. By the end of eight years in Europe and my doctoral work, I had lost most of that Southern accent—or so I thought. However, teaching in Decatur, Georgia for ten years revived some of that melodious, dripping-with-honey, filled with diphthongs type of speech. When my academic journey took me to the Midwest, my speech became a novelty. This background is important for what comes next.

A revered senior pastor and chaplain to the university and theological school where I taught was a man of great wisdom and respect. He and his wife did not have biological children, and they poured their lives into students on campus. The chaplain often mentored the graduate students in the theology school or seminary, especially those invested in church ministry. There was one most outstanding seminary student who had leadership responsibilities on campus and was such a gracious person to all students, including international and undergraduate students. Unbeknownst to most of us at the time, this student leader on campus went through a very hard time, perhaps "a dark night of the soul." He concealed it, but the chaplain knew and met with him to give counsel.

We then received the news that this beloved seminary student had attempted suicide in a gruesome way, had not succeeded, and was near death in a hospital. He lingered, but did not survive. A meeting was called of all senior administrations. The chaplain was included. I was invited as professor of pastoral care. The meeting did not start right away because the chaplain was in so much excruciating pain—physically, mentally, spiritually. As is common after a suicide, he flagellated himself with statements of "should have," "could have," "didn't think he would do it." He was in more than shock and disbelief. He was in shame, guilt, and deepening despair. It was as if his spirit was disintegrating before us.

Something overcame me. In the most authoritative tone of voice, firm and well-projected, with no trace of the South, I said his name and declared: "[name], God would **not** have you carry that burden." There was silence and gravitas in the room. There was a hushed quiet over the gathered administrators followed by a shift in the demeanor, spirit, and carriage of the chaplain of the university. Pastors, rabbis, imams, chaplains, and ministers of all sorts reading this story will know that this authority comes to us from our Higher Power or Source. It is an authoritative utterance or word "given" to us.

Just as a physician or surgeon assembles a team, so did I in the situation described above. I did not wait to clear what I wanted to do through the officials at the university, HR, the president or deans. I acted as I had been trained to do as a pastoral counselor and psychotherapist, as a minister ordained by the PCUSA. I called for help. I contacted a psychiatrist who was a member of the church I attended. The fallout over campus was so extensive that I thought of the Civil War images of the wounded flung all over the battlefield, writhing in pain, desperate for a stretcher or aid. The psychiatrist told me to call the American Red Cross. This suggestion was something I had never thought of as a resource. I called, got an immediate response, and the next day the American Red Cross assembled the finest psychiatrists, psychologists, licensed professional counselors, marriage and family therapists, licensed clinical social workers that the Midwestern city had to offer. All of these professionals were on a volunteer, call-up, emergency list with the Red Cross. They came quickly. The children in the seminary village had their own therapist; the spouses in the village had theirs; the seminary students were divided into groups; the Native American seminary students wanted their own counselor; and so it went. To this day, I am grateful for the team of healers that came. I am thankful for "the authority invested in me" at ordination and by the Ultimate Authority I serve.

HEALING USING EVERY MEANS OF CURE

Chrysostom wrote that physicians of the body do not cure in one manner only. The analogy is that physicians of the soul engage in healing using every means of cure. Physicians of the soul can always grow more sensitive to approaches to pastoral and spiritual care from a variety of practices, both Christian and non. Examples of these are Native American traditional healing, homeopathy, reflexology, meditation, trauma-informed yoga, energy medicine, and other forms of alternative healing—alternative to modern scientific medicine. This list is not exhaustive, by any means. It is encouraging that mainstream medicine as well as insurance companies are now listing several of these practices as other accepted forms of pain management. With an understanding and an undergirding of wholistic healing, we as physicians of the soul also listen, learn, and adapt our spiritual care practices to meet the needs and the *soul wounds* of the human beings that the Creator places in our path. In what follows, we will look at a variety of these nontraditional care practices.

COMMUNITY

We should never forget that the community can be a means of care and of cure. In the case below, the community is a theological school. Community, in this sense, could also be a seminary, a church, a synagogue, a congregation, or another aggregate of caring people. All of these groups have the potential to form a caring web around one of their members.

With permission, I use Naomi's story from 2021 during the pandemic. When Covid-19 shut down travel, some of our international students at Perkins School of Theology, Southern Methodist University (SMU), Dallas, faced extraordinary challenges and isolation. I had two students in my class from Kenya with these circumstances. As professors went into a Hy-Flex mode of teaching, I announced at the beginning of each semester during Covid-19 that our school had resources to help with home internet insecurity or lack of home equipment. This was a reiteration of a message sent out by the dean to make sure all students could continue classes. Naomi approached me privately after the second week of class. What she had heard was: we had resources to offer. She helped me to understand that the university Food Pantry had been closed since the outbreak of Covid-19. Although the food pantry during the pandemic gave her a hundred-dollar monthly gift voucher for food, it did not stretch to feed herself and her two children. Her support had been cut off from Kenya due to the critical illness of her working parent.

As the community became aware of Naomi's circumstances, everyone jumped into action. Colleagues provided money for food; a student bought warm clothing when the winter blizzard paralyzed the city of Dallas in February; our dean took Naomi and another student from Kenya grocery shopping during the ice storm. A woman whom I had not seen nor talked to in five years sent me a large check to use for "a cause on my heart." This woman lived in another state and had no idea of this situation. She was prompted while in prayer. Faculty began to advocate for university assistance.

At the end of the semester, Naomi approached me with an amazing result. Unbeknownst to me, Naomi had suffered from a severe skin rash for months. She had always worn a jacket with long sleeves in class accompanied by a head scarf and a mask for Covid-19 protection. I did not realize what all this clothing was covering. She first turned to the SMU student health center. The rash over the upper portion of her body and arms did not clear up. The health center referred her to specialists, primarily dermatologists and allergists, but the treatments were ineffective. And yet, as she began to experience caring connectedness from members of our community, support from as far away as Nashville, her rash disappeared. She attributed the healing of her rash to the "mothering" she had received from those in the community whose hands had been extended to her.

FAMILY SYSTEMS THEORY

In the course of teaching family systems theory, I have also witnessed instances of healing. Family systems theory is an approach or a lens to understanding the dynamics of families and other systems like the church. This lens through which to view yourself is not only a way to freedom but to health and healing. Pastoral care in its traditional form focused on the individual (Sigmund Freud, Alfred Adler, Rollo May, Victor Frankl, Abraham Maslow), but pastoral care in recent decades views individuals in open social systems which are constantly undergoing structural transformations.

We live amidst many systems. They surround us: circulatory, respiratory, neurological, ecological, computer, electrical, political, legal, criminal justice, and many more. Yet, the system we encounter at our earliest age is familial whether through birth, adoption, or fosterage. It is this system that impacts us greatly. Family systems theory allows each person to see the role they played in the family in which they were born, fostered, or adopted. This is called the *family of origin*. When we recognize the expectations, the limitations, etc., that were placed upon us in our family of origin, we can make choices to change, a process called self-differentiation. Our position among siblings can also affect our roles we adopt; with self-awareness, we can learn to be a more authentic self. Much personal healing can occur as we gain insight and seek to become the person God has created us to be.

One graduate student, Elsie, who had been abandoned as a baby by her birth mother had scant information on her family of origin. A requirement of the family systems course was to diagram a family tree or *genogram*. This student resisted doing this for several months, even when she had to turn in a blank piece of paper for her family tree. All she had on that paper was her grandmother who raised her. She hated her birth mother who had cast her aside as an infant. The student refused to talk with her grandmother about her mother or any other family members. I asked her to put down just a few names, but she adamantly resisted any knowledge of her birth family outside of her beloved grandmother.

Imagine my surprise one Sunday a year later when she invited me to speak in her AME (African Methodist Episcopal) church in downtown Dallas. She introduced me to her congregation, Agape Temple AME, as her pastoral care professor. First, she told her congregation that I had lowered her grade in family systems because she didn't have much information. There was an audible rumbling of disapproval. I sank low into my seat near the pulpit. Then, she asked her mother—and aunt—and cousins—to stand up in the congregation. It turned out this student had flown out to California, located her frail mother in a destitute situation, and brought her back to Dallas. This student cared for her sick mother during what was to be the last year of her mother's life. Mother and daughter were together at the last. As a friend remarked, "Forgiveness is very freeing." Most of all, God gave her forgiveness and peace. By the way, I raised Elsie's genogram grade to an A+.

Elsie went on to earn a Doctor of Ministry degree. On the night before graduation, there is a banquet for all graduates and their families. To my amazement, there was one table that was packed full of people. It was Elsie's table. She was surrounded by aunts and cousins who had driven in to celebrate. Through Elsie's family systems work, this family had found each other. That blank piece of paper that held only one circle, grandmother, was now filling up.

Elsie became an acclaimed preacher and seasoned pastor. She was diagnosed with terminal cancer at the pinnacle of her career. She ministered as long as she could. When she came close to her last days, her church ministered to her. Her long-lost biological sister drove up from Houston to Dallas to tend to her along with her parishioners, seminary faculty, and ministerial colleagues. The head of Faith Hospice told me she had never seen any client hold on so long. We decided Elsie wanted to be with her extended family just a little longer, making up for those years she had no one but her grandmother to put on her genogram. Her church members camped out on the floor of her home; some prayed, some sang hymns, some rubbed her arms with lotion. Elsie died of fourth-stage cancer, but the bitterness of abandonment and the soul-biting sense of being unwanted had long since been healed. It was a Homecoming of Healing.

More and more pastors, pastoral counselors, therapists, licensed professional counselors, and clinical pastoral educators are using family systems theory as a lens for the type of healing demonstrated in Elsie's journey.

YOGA

At a dinner in Pittsburgh, I was seated next to Joanne Spence, MA, E-RYT 500, C-IAYT who is author of *Trauma-Informed Yoga: A Toolbox for Therapists.* It was only after the initial pleasantries at a mutual friend's retirement party that Joanne and I realized that we were both deeply interested in healing. Joanne is a certified yoga therapist and a former social worker. She has taught yoga in a variety of settings: hospitals, schools, prisons, churches, and street corners. Her specialty is working with children and adults experiencing chronic pain, depression, insomnia, anxiety, ADHD, and trauma. It was that last word that caught my attention.

In the Prologue to *The Body Keeps Score*, Bessel Van der Kolk, MD, offers statistics from the American Journal of Preventive Medicine. She writes,

> Research by the Centers of Disease Control and Prevention has shown that one in five Americans was sexually molested as a child; one in four was beaten by a parent to the point of a mark being left on their body; and one in three couples engages in physical violence. A quarter of us grew up with alcoholic relatives, and one in eight witnessed their mother being beaten or hit.[23]

When I first started teaching "Pastoral Care of Women" in 1986, the statistics were one of four women were raped, one in three women and children were beaten in their homes. I would ask seminary students to imagine those numbers in their congregation and be sensitive with material chosen for worship.

Joanne Spence came into my Pastoral Self-Care class by ZOOM. The majority of the students in class had never experienced yoga. While seated in our chairs, we practiced gentle movement and breathing, visualization and meditation. We learned about the ventral vagal circuit which "provides us with a sense of safety and connection in the context of relationships."[24] At the end of class, Joanne had us imagine tool belts around our waist, and we were encouraged to put the breathing and relaxation techniques we learned in the pockets of the tool belt—there when needed. The next week a student came to me after class and said she had applied some of these techniques at the onset of an anxiety attack before a test in another class. She was suffering from an anxiety disorder. She had enough in her tool belt to quell the attack. This is not to imply she was healed from her anxiety disorder, but it does indicate that she was making a small step toward healing.

PSYCHOANALYSIS

Orna Guralnik is a psychologist who works with individuals and couples. Since the mid-twentieth century, there have been changes in the dynamics and conversations of couples, profound changes caused by progressive movements like #MeToo, Black Lives Matter (BLM), and trans rights. Guralnik writes, "In my practice, I've found engaging with these progressive movements has led to deep changes in our psyches. My patients, regardless of political affiliation, are incorporating the message of social movements into the very structure of their being."[25] Implicit biases, generational trauma, the relevance of class, privilege, skin color, and race in marriages and partnerships are being acknowledged and sometimes fought over in her counseling sessions with couples. "As a collective we appear to be coming around to the idea that bigger social forces run through us, animating us and pitting us against one another, whatever our conscious intentions. To invert a truism, the political is personal."[26] For her and other therapists, a deeper level of honesty has erupted in couples' counseling, bringing a novel understanding of social factors and the impact of systems. Guralnik's work is made easier as her clients become aware of unconscious complicity and unconscious forces in their social systems. When these systems are different, acknowledgement of the radical *otherness of the partner* is a movement forward and a challenge. Guralnik works as a therapist to encourage cessation of guilt and defensiveness, and acceptance of multiple perspectives. "Love is ultimately measured by people's capacity to see and care about the other person as they are; succeeding in this effort is how people grow in relationships."[27] Again, this is only one more example of current ways healers, in this case a psychoanalyst, are attempting to find new means of curing people.

BINDING THE WOUNDS

In the *Tractate Sanhedrin*, chapter 11, of the Babylonian Talmud, the Messiah sits at the gate of the city, binding up one wound at a time, leaving some wounds exposed in the event he should be called away. Thus, the concept of the wounded minister and the healing minister can be combined.[28]

Binding and unbinding and binding. The wounds need to be bound. The focus never seems to fall on those surrounding the Messiah, the poor covered with wounds. Their wounds are all exposed, and they are obviously not in the same rhythm as the Messiah. They are not in any condition to get up and be of service.

Who are these people? Are they poor in spirit? In assets? In bodily vitality? In health? Do they have "diseases of the soul"? We have no clue except they are extensively impaired, covered with wounds, scabs, and open sores. They are acting inappropriately, nonsensically, irrationally. They remain sitting, perhaps unable to stand or move. They are not healed enough to be able to respond if needed. Yet the Messiah responds. A physician of the soul responds, especially attuned to soul-wounds.

Religious leaders, pastoral counselors, ministers and other helping professionals are being increasingly sought after for treatment of soul-wounds. For example, following a rape, a pelvic exam would be a medical procedure. If there are tears in the vaginal area, bruising, cuts, or other injuries, this also would be handled by the physicians of the body. After a trauma such as this, it is common to have the emotion of fear, for example, which contributes to a startle reflex. There is a complex of emotions which can be tended to by physicians of the mind such as a psychiatrist or clinical psychologist. However, on the deepest level, the soul is penetrated in such a brutal way that a sense of worth, dignity, safety, and a belief of being a beloved of God are in question.[29] Veterans of wars are treated not only for physical injuries sustained, but for a mental reality of Post-Traumatic-Stress Syndrome that can trigger memories. For those who have been raised on "thou shall not kill" and on the dignity of all people, the scarring and after-effect of killing is an anguish of the soul. Native American therapists and psychologists are teaching us "the Native idea of historical trauma involves [understanding] that the trauma occurred in the soul or spirit, and was and is understood as soul wound."[30] Trauma studies are illustrating clearly the interconnection of body-mind-soul. For that, we need more than one remedy.

MORE THAN ONE REMEDY

How do physicians of the soul function for coping with dis-eases of the soul? Pastoral presence, attentive listening, learning from others as living human documents, following the lead of patients, listening for their clues and cues, claiming holy spaces, asking for help when we need it, remembering we are not alone. In the words of Chrysostom, "Bestowing attention and tender care, by trying every means of amendment, in imitation of the best physicians, for neither do they cure in one manner only, but when they see the wound not yield to the first remedy, they add another, and after again another." However, as the case of Naomi illustrates, in addition to all that has been said, we cannot underplay the role of community. A vital query, especially in crisis, is this: How do physicians of the soul partner with physicians of the mind and of the body in the midst of catastrophe and trauma? How do I function uniquely as a physician of the soul with those suffering Post-Traumatic Stress, soul-wounding, the legacy of historical trauma? I recall the words attributed to Hippocrates, from whom we will hear more in chapter three: "In order to cure the human body, it is necessary to have a knowledge of the whole of things."[31]

Crisis has many faces: scarred, afraid, diseased, shattered, hungry, thirsty, mutilated, or covered with a rash. Our role as practical and pastoral theologians is to care, to accompany, to attend, and—in some cases—to cure. We will not only look at various methods of healing, but imagine ways healers of the body, mind, and soul can better work as a team. Jason Sion Mokhtarian has looked at medicine in the Talmud and concluded, "Medicine in the Talmud consists of both natural and supernatural therapies that operated between magic and science . . . . For the rabbis, magical and empirical medicine, or natural and supernatural etiologies and therapies, were not mutually exclusive or even dichotomous so much as they were fused together in the real world."[32] Today, physicians of the soul operate among miracle and medicine—and mystery.

THE CASE OF ANNE O'CONNELL: PART 2

Focus on the numerous players in this true case: extended family, priest, physicians, nurses, hospital chaplain.

Anne was at Mayo Clinic with her parents. She had been diagnosed with a sarcoma, a tumor on her right fibula, just below the knee. The leg would have to be amputated above the knee. Anne's father asked Dr. F. H. Sims if he could save Anne's life. Dr. Sims hesitated and said he would try, but her cancer was a grade four.

At this point an amazing intervention happened. Anne described her "little Irish mother" going up to her X-ray and looking at her right leg. She bravely asked: "Could you do a resection to save her leg?" Dr. Sims looked at the X-ray and admitted he had never done that surgery before. He would consider whether he could do it or not. Anne commented: "At that moment, looking at my dear mother, I thought how inspiring this act of love was." They met with Dr. Sims again and discussed a resection. Then, they contacted Father Pius who felt strongly that the amputation should not be done. The monks were praying. Anne and her family returned to many phone calls of concern and prayers. She and her parents returned to Rochester on April 8, 1976, to St. Mary's Hospital. For her surgery on April 9, 1976, they were all wondering what tomorrow would bring. They put Anne's life in God's hands. Her mother brought in the hospital chaplain who anointed her with holy oil. Although Anne had already been anointed by Father Pius, "the sacrament is also given for God's strength and courage."

On April 9, 1976, her surgery was to start at 8:00, but was delayed because another patient needed emergency surgery. "I totally accepted this. I received many hugs and good luck wishes from many family members." Aunts, uncles, her parents, and her brothers were there to support Anne. Then, the surgical nurse came at 11:15 to take her to the elevator, down to surgery. "I was emotional and had some tears. The nurse said, 'Why are you crying?'"

NOTES

1   Robert Dykstra, *Images of Pastoral Care: Classic Readings* (Danvers, MA: Chalice Press, 2005). This treasure trove of metaphors for understanding pastoral care contains nineteen images from the history of the discipline. However, physician of the soul was overlooked.

2   Jennifer Barry, *Bishops in Flight: Exile and Displacement in Late Antiquity* (Oakland, CA: University of California Press, 2019), 93.

3   Elizabeth A. Clark, "John Chrysostom and the 'Subintroductae'" *Church History* 46 (1977): 171–85. Chrysostom along with Athanasius of Alexandria, Jerome, Eusebius of Emesa, and Gregory of Nyssa felt that lust could alter the relationship.

4 Aideen Hartney, *John Chrysostom and the Transformation of the City* (London: Duckworth, 2004).

5 Barry, *Bishops in Flight*, 93.

6 Courtney Wilson Van Veller, "Paul's Therapy of the Soul: A New Approach to John Chrysostom and Anti-Judaism" (PhD diss., Boston University, 2015). Van Veller argues that in Chrysostom's sermons on Acts and the Pauline Epistles, Chrysostom writes with a subtle anti-Judaism that views Jewish difference as a disease that even Paul's oratorical and sermonic surgery could not remove. I am retrieving this term in order to use it in a vastly different way; however, I want to acknowledge the deplorable anti-Jewish rhetoric in which this term is occasionally found and call out its impropriety.

7 Chrysostom, "Homily III," 62.

8 Chrysostom, "Homily IX," 158

9 Chrysostom, "Homily XXIX," 511.

10 Chrysostom, "Homily VI," 125.

11 Chrysostom, "Homily VII," 140.

12 Chrysostom, "Homily VII," 139.

13 Chrysostom, "Homily VII," 126.

14 Chrysostom, "Homily VII," 143.

15 Chrysostom, "Homily VII," 126.

16 Informal Interview with addiction therapist, Charter Peachford Hospital, Atlanta, GA, 1988.

17 Informal Interview with addiction therapist, at Charter Peachford Hospital, 1988.

18 Gordon J. Hilsman, "The Unconsciously Hidden: Potential Drinking Problems in the General Hospital" in *Confrontation in Spiritual Care: An Anthology for Clinical Caregivers*, eds. Hilsman and Sandra Walker (Olympia: Summit Bay Press, 2022), 29–43. Hilsman, as chaplain at Presbyterian St. Luke's Medical Center in Chicago, used a calmer, gentler approach with patients whom he suspected were suffering from alcoholism. His example in this chapter centers on a young man, hospitalized after a vehicle crash. The ER report showed he had been drinking. Hilsman hoped to convince him to go into treatment for alcoholism and used a softer approach than what I experienced at Charter Peachford Hospital, Addictive Disease Unit.

19 Gordon J. Hilsman and Sandra Walker eds., *Confrontation in Spiritual Care: An Anthology for Clinical Caregivers* (Olympia, WA: Summit Bay Press, 2022), 175.

20 The full and literal translation from the Greek text is this: "Accordingly when thou seest an enemy of the truth, wait on (him), take care of (him), lead (him) back to virtue, by showing forth an excellent life, by applying the word without accusation, bestowing attention with authority and standing with the authority of a physician, a protector, ones who shows care." This is my own translation from the original Greek text of Joannis Chrysostomi. Homily XXIX, Matt. IX.1,2, p. 517. [1248] and [1249] in Homilies on the Gospel of St.Matthew (I-XLV), St. John Chrysostom, Excerpter From A Select Library of the Nicene and Post-Nicene Fathers of the Christian Church, ed. Paul A Boer, Sr., (Veritatis Splendor Publications, 2012).

21 Lindsey Johnson Edwards, "Medicine and the Market: The Misenchantment of Modernity" (paper, Southern Methodist University, 2023), 2.

22 J. Frederick Holper, "What does it mean to be ordained?" Presbyterianmission.org, Presbyterian Church USA), 2023, https://tinyurl.com/2b9xf596.

23 Bessel Van Der Kolk, MD. *The Body Keeps Score: Brain, Mind, and Body in the Healing of Trauma* (New York: Penguin Books, 2014), 1. Statistics cited from V. Felitti, et al. "Relationship of Childhood Abuse and Household Dysfunction to Many of the Leading Causes of Death in Adults: The Adverse Childhood Experiences (ACE) Study." *American Journal of Preventive Medicine* 14 (1998): 245–58.

24 Spence, Joanne, *Trauma-Informed Yoga: A Toolbox for Therapists* (Eau Claire, WI: PESI Publishing, 2021), 38.

25 Orna Guralnik, "I'm a Couples Therapist: Something New is Happening in Relationships," in *The New York Times Magazine* 16.5 (2023): 37.

26 Guralnik, "I'm a Couples Therapist: Something New is Happening in Relationships," 37.

27 Guralnik, "I'm a Couples Therapist: Something New is Happening in Relationships," 37.

28 Jeanne Stevenson-Moessner, "The Impaired Healer," (unpublished paper, Southern Methodist University, 2023).

29 At Perkins School of Theology, I offer an elective on "Sexual and Domestic Violence." The class is composed of men and women training for ministry. In addition to the classroom experience of lectures, discussions, readings, videos, speakers, the students actually train **in** a domestic violence program (Genesis) and in a

rape crisis center (Texas Health Presbyterian Hospital's Center for SAFE Healing). This has a twofold purpose. The student as pastor may be called to accompany a parishioner to either of these types of healing places. The students also learn to make connections with such resources when they **first** settle into an appointment or parish. Again, this is an elective course.

30 Eduardo Duran, *Healing the Soul Wound* (New York: Teachers College Press, 2019), 10.

31 This quote is attributed to Dr. Yatish Agarwal, *The World Within: Symptoms and Remedies of the Mind* (New Delhi: Rajkamal Books, 2004), 174.

32 Jason Sion Mokhtarian *Medicine in the Talmud: Natural and Supernatural Therapies between Magic and Science* (Oakland: University of California Press, 2022), 113–14.

THREE

Soulful Medicine and Soul-Filled Ministry

A college student once asked Dr. Howard Thurman for advice. The student was at a crossroads and was trying to decide whether to pursue a career in medicine, ministry, or law. Dr. Thurman agreed that all three choices were worthy. However, Thurman steered the student in a different direction: "Don't ask yourself what the world needs. Ask yourself what makes you come alive, and go do that, because what the world needs is people who have come alive."[1]

Professional caregiving is usually a vocation in which one feels fully alive. Granted there are times of frustration and compassion fatigue. Yet, it is fairly likely that those in chaplaincy, ministry, palliative care, hospice, all forms of caregiving including medical caregiving, have the gifts of mercy and hospitality; these are biblical gifts which we cannot conjure up. These gifts are bestowed on us, and if this is true, it is our freedom to receive these. It is possible that the art of healing requires gifts such as these.

SOULFUL MEDICINE

Soulful is an adjective that has often be used to describe music expressing deep emotions and coming from the essence of the musician's being. Examples can be found in James Cone's *The Spirituals and the Blues,* a presentation of these two anchoring art forms of the African-American experience.[2] Soulful is considered passionate. In music, that passion can often convey lament, liberation, and identity: "Black music is the music of the soul, the music of the black psyche renewing itself for living and being."[3]

Soulful medicine comes from a very deep place in the soul that is capable of deep emotions, responsive to suffering, and committed to actions of virtue. It is in line with the Hippocratic Oath. The classic version contains the following statement: "In purity and holiness I will pass my life and practice my art [*techne*]."[4] The word *techne* is translated as art and science.

Dr. Curtis, associate medical director of Laguna Honda Hospital in San Francisco, is an example of this. In *God's Hotel,* Dr. Victoria Sweet learns about soulful medicine from Dr. Curtis. He had taken a year off after college to go to India to study yoga, Sanskrit, and Indian spirituality and Indian medicine. After medical school, he offered time-costly caring at Laguna Honda, the last "almshouse" for the sick and poor. Sweet described him as a man "who saw further and deeper than the rest of us"[5] and exhibited what the Greeks called *entheos* or "having a god within."[6] While making rounds among the stroke patients in rehabilitation, he noticed one patient who was overdue for discharge. Approaching the patient waiting in a wheelchair, he asked why he was not discharged now that he could walk. The patient replied that he had no shoes although the hospital had ordered special shoes for him. The hospital had been waiting three months for Medicaid to approve them. Dr. Curtis asked for his shoe size, went immediately to Walmart, found shoes for $16.99, and returned shortly thereafter to the hospital. Sweet admits that for the first time she understood what Dr. Francis Peabody said to the 1927 graduating medical class at Harvard: "The secret in the care of the patient is in caring for the patient."[7] Not just caring about the patient but caring for the patient means doing the little things. This could be offering a sip of water, wiping spittle off the chin, or buying shoes from Walmart.[8]

THE HIPPOCRATIC OATH

At the time my father and his elder twin brothers graduated from the University of Tennessee medical school, they would have taken the Hippocratic Oath, an oath to practice their art in a holy manner. Today, there are several versions and adaptations of the Oath, originally written in Iconic Greek. There is no historical certainty that Hippocrates himself wrote the Oath. It was written around 400 BCE and opens with an appeal to gods and goddesses. In *The Hippocratic Oath and the Ethics of Medicine*, Stephen Miles summarizes the intent: "On closer inspection, its 400 words sweep from the mythic origin of medicine along a professional ancestry and point to the future judgment on the profession. The Oath proposes principles and rules for medicine."[9] The undergirding proposition was "to do no harm," a phrase that has come to characterize the Oath itself and the medicinal art it aims to protect. Some medical schools today use more modern versions that are written in the vernacular; some schools have a shortened version or cease to use it at all. The classic version contains the following statement: "In purity and holiness I will pass my life and practice my art [*techne*]." The words in the Oath for "purity and holiness" are the Greek words (in adverbial form): ἁγνῶς is translated "full of religious awe," while ὁσίως is translated as "devoutly," "in a manner pleasing to the gods," and "in a holy manner."[10] The appeal to the gods of the Oath were Apollo, Apollo's son Asclepius, and the daughters of Apollo and Epione (also a healer). The daughters were Hygieia (goddess of health, hygiene, and preventive care) and Panacea (goddess of remedies).[11] Health, hygiene, and preventive care became an essential element in healing as seen in the protocol of the first woman to receive a medical degree as a physician in the United States, Dr. Elizabeth Blackwell (1821–1920), and of nurse Florence Nightingale, "The Lady with the Lamp" (1820–1920), who implemented hygiene practices during the Crimean War and saved countless soldiers.

From its creation, the Oath was framed in a sacred manner. Throughout history, the gods and goddesses invoked for health and healing vary, reflecting specific time periods and historical contexts, but the thread that binds the creation of the oath all the way to the present day is the understanding that medicine is a sacred trust. The names of our Divine Power and Wholly Other may be numerous but physicians of mind, body, and soul carry a sacrosanct duty to heal and to do no harm. This duty is often too much for physicians to bear as much remains out of their control, thus the divine becomes the one whom physicians call upon.

The concept of a sacred trust is coupled at this juncture with a calling. "In the first century, Scribonius Largus referred to Hippocrates as the founder of the 'calling [of medicine].'"[12] In summary, our interconnection of physicians of body-mind-soul recalls the common features of our vocational birth cord (*funiculus umbilicalis*) as healers: our work is sacred; our work is a calling.

PHYSICIAN OF SOULS

THE HIPPOCRATIC OATH:
CLASSICAL VERSION[13]

I swear by Apollo Physician and Asclepius and Hygieia and Panaceia and all the gods and goddesses, making them my witnesses, that I will fulfill according to my ability and judgment this oath and this covenant:

To hold him who has taught me this art as equal to my parents and to live my life in partnership with him, and if he is in need of money to give him a share of mine, and to regard his offspring as equal to my brothers in male lineage and to teach them this art—if they desire to learn it—without fee and covenant; to give a share of precepts and oral instruction and all the other learning to my sons and to the sons of him who has instructed me and to pupils who have signed the covenant and have taken an oath according to the medical law, but no one else.

I will apply dietetic measures for the benefit of the sick according to my ability and judgment; I will keep them from harm and injustice.

I will neither give a deadly drug to anybody who asked for it, nor will I make a suggestion to this effect. Similarly, I will not give to a woman an abortive remedy. **In purity and holiness, I will guard my life and my art.**

I will not use the knife, not even on sufferers from stone, but will withdraw in favor of such men as are engaged in this work.

Whatever houses I may visit, I will come for the benefit of the sick, remaining free of all intentional injustice, of all mischief and in particular of sexual relations with both female and male persons, be they free or slaves.

What I may see or hear in the course of the treatment or even outside of the treatment in regard to the life of men, which on no account one must spread abroad, I will keep to myself, holding such things shameful to be spoken about.

If I fulfill this oath and do not violate it, may it be granted to me to enjoy life and art, being honored with fame among all men for all time to come; if I transgress it and swear falsely, may the opposite of all this be my lot.

THE NECESSITY FOR THE OATH AND THE CREDO

Why do we need an oath in the practice of medicine? Is the same true for religion? We are aware now more than ever with advanced media and news outlets in the twenty-first century that a person practicing medicine or religion can do grave harm. I was convinced of this necessity of an oath or credo during my first year of teaching after returning to the United States.[14] I was at a PCUSA seminary in the South as an adjunct. I taught a course that no one else there was teaching at that time: pastoral care of women. I knew to choose the books carefully because I knew students were on a tight budget. One of the textbooks was titled *Is Nothing Sacred? When Sex Invades the Pastoral Relationship* by Marie Fortune.[15] This was 1992, and the book had just come out in hardback. I put in down as required reading. It was one detailed case study, a true story, of a male pastor who sexually abused women in his study, hid the scandal for years, and almost destroyed his congregation when it was discovered. The maneuvers and secret mechanisms that covered up this pattern of violation of vulnerable women was exposed, analyzed, and condemned by Rev. Marie Fortune. She also laid out not only the legal machinery that was put into place, but the struggle of the entire congregation to exist.

As I reflected at the end of the semester, I thought I had made a mistake in making this book required reading. It was an expensive hardback. After all, it was only one case study, albeit in great detail. Had I wasted the students' money? It beleaguered me. Two years later, in 1994, at a continuing education event on campus, a graduate who had taken this class stopped me. She was in a Southern state in a small town with two churches, Presbyterian and Baptist. She was the Presbyterian pastor. On a Saturday afternoon while she was in the kitchen of the manse, there was a timid knock on the door. She opened it and was surprised to see the wife of the Baptist minister, looking uneasy and very stressed. Over a hot cup of tea, the wife of the Baptist minister finally told her reason for coming. She found out that her husband was having sexual intercourse with some of his counselees, women of the church. Then she laid out the scenario, and it was exactly the same as in *Is Nothing Sacred? When Sex Invades the Pastoral Relationship*! Then she told the PCUSA pastor: "I knew I could come to you because I knew you would believe me." She did, and she knew what to do. At the continuing education event, she approached me and said: "I knew I was prepared for that moment." The news since 1994 has been filled with scandals such as this, involving physicians of the soul (pastors, religious leaders) who have seriously wounded those in their care, those who trusted them.

They have done grave harm, perhaps irreparable. There are equal amounts of accounts of physicians' abuse of patients, for example, the scandal of Dr. Larry Nassar, now a convicted rapist. As team doctor of the USA Gymnastics Team and as professor at Michigan State University, he sexually manipulated and assaulted hundreds of children and young women.

The Oath set boundaries for physicians of the body just as those of use in ministry take oaths at our ordination. The Oath attributed to Hippocrates reads: "Whatever houses I may visit, I will come for the benefit of the sick, remaining free of all intentional injustice, of all mischief and in particular of sexual relations with both female and male persons, be they free or slaves." There is a clear obligation to the teachers of the physician as well as to their offspring. There is promise to withhold deadly drugs and abortive remedies. If not trained as a surgeon, the knife (scalpel) would not be used. Confidentiality was to be kept. The Oath is an ethic of caring, some of which is applicable not only to medicine but to ministry. Ethics provide both boundaries and accountability.

What was admired about Hippocrates was not so much his knowledge of anatomy and physiology. According to G.E.R. Lord, the admiration stemmed from "the example he set of the doctor's devotion and concern for his patients, and of his uprightness and discretion in his dealings with them . . . While most of the anatomical, physiological, and pathological doctrines in the Hippocratic writings have long been superseded, the ideal of the selfless, dedicated and compassionate doctor they present has lost none of its relevance."[16] Hippocratic medicine is meant to be holistic. Holistic medicine involves the treatment of the whole person with attention paid to cultural, mental, and social factors, rather than a focus on the symptoms of the disease or illness. It is adaptable and appropriate for numerous approaches to modern-day medicine. Hippocrates is favored by homeopathists, naturopaths, chiropractors, herbalists, and osteopaths "as the founder of the ideals that underlie their own approaches to health, disease, and healing."[17]

Hippocratic medicine concerns the whole patient. Holism was rooted in Greek cultural values. For example, the Greeks disliked dissection of bodies. There were no autopsies. Students learned through their teachers. There were no hospitals or medical schools. Care would have been given at the bedside of actual patients. Granted it was surface anatomy. Yet, the Hippocratic approach was the prototype of modern primary care. "The Hippocratic doctor needed to know his patient thoroughly: what his social, economic, and familial circumstances were, how he lived, what he usually ate and drank, whether he had travelled or not, whether slave or free, tendencies to disease."[18] It was a pivotal moment in the history of medicine when Hippocratic treatises established that disease was not associated with the anger of gods. Medicine could be associated with the physical causes. In an ironic way, the development of medicine as a natural study and science could have lead to the subsequent bifurcation of medicine and religion.

THE CAREGIVER'S CREDO

John Chrysostom was a moral theologian and concerned with right actions undergirded by a moral code. I have taken his term *physician of souls* and developed a credo, a statement of beliefs that guide actions. The creed is in tune with the demands of the twenty-first century in theological schools today. The credo aligns itself with the need to include personal aspects such as the culture of the individual and the necessity to prevent exploitation, degradation, humiliation, and stereotyping of the suffering individual. With the increasing attention to trauma, this credo offers safety in approach and treatment.

Physicians of souls also need a credo, and I offer one as a model for further credos. My model includes these beliefs and convictions:

a. recognition of the interconnection of body-mind-soul-culture;

b. a stance that no one deserves to be exploited, violated, degraded, or suppressed;

c. a resistance to a culture that does so;

d. an awareness that the body is a place where God can dwell; this awareness results in actions that respect that holy place;

e. a belief that the worth of a person is not based on contour, color, creed, or capabilities;

f. a commitment to the importance of community in the healing process;

g. conviction about the critical role of the "holding environment" of the hospital;

h. an understanding of a patient's essential need to feel valued and to be heard;

i. an affirmation of both rituals of medicine and rituals in healing.[19]

Recognition of the interconnection of body-mind-soul-culture

At a Native American conference on "Healing with Dignity" at Perkins School of Theology, I heard the story of Jim Labelle with the Boarding School

Healing Coalition for Native Americans. Jim told his own story in a documentary that we watched. He had been snatched from his mother at age eight, put in a Canadian boarding school, stripped of his name and language, and cried himself to sleep each boyhood night along with other little boys who had been given new English names. This was a significant yet sorrowful aspect of his spiritual journey. Shortly thereafter, I heard a prestigious visiting scholar mention the phrase "our common spiritual journey" just once too often. In the question and answer time, I raised my hand and challenged that notion. It was at that moment that I knew deeply that we as humans do not have a common spiritual journey. I was not torn away from my family at eight, told I could not speak my language or use my Native name, put in strange clothes, and severed from my culture like Jim Labelle. We may all have a spiritual journey but it is not common. Physicians of the soul are called to recognize the lasting effect culture has on the mind-body-soul/spiritual journey and to acknowledge the role culture has in healing the whole person.

Psychologist Eduardo Duran calls attention to the importance of the **culture** of the patient. His research and work have centered on Indigenous people. New healing narratives are surfacing as the world view of Indigenous people are being understood by medical doctors and therapists: "Historical narcissism (the belief that one's own system of thinking must be used to validate other cultural belief systems) continues to be an issue in the relationship between Indigenous people and those who hold power in the academic and clinical life-world."[20] Much of his research centers on culturally transmitted trauma.

Native Americans have taught us that culturally transmitted trauma goes seven generations back.

If it is not dealt with in the current generation, the trauma will be passed on to the following seven generations of descendants. The urgency for reconciliation, restitution, and forgiveness is imperative and crucial among the current generation for this reason.[21] Native Americans I have met do not want to saddle their children and their children's children with the raw trauma and pain.

A stance that no one deserves to be exploited, violated, degraded, or suppressed

The Hippocratic Oath and the Caregiver's Oath make a firm stand against the exploitation of those suffering. Stories have surfaced of the suffering of people, for example, African-American women who were sterilized and used for scientific and social experiments. The most famous and well-documented is that of Henrietta Lacks (1920–1951) who entered Johns Hopkins Hospital in 1951 with cervical cancer. A biopsy was taken, and the cells cultured. Her cells were unique and were developed into the *HeLa* cell line for medical research; they were labeled "immortal" because they rapidly reproduced and divided repeatedly, allowing for extended and breakthrough cellular research. Henrietta was never asked for permission; her family was not notified of this ongoing use of Henrietta's cells until many years after her death.[22] Recently, the Associated Press confirmed that the sterilization of Indigenous women has not ended in Canada. "Decades after many other rich countries stopped forcibly sterilizing Indigenous women, numerous activists, doctors, politicians and at least five class-action lawsuits allege the practice has not ended in Canada."[23]

A resistance to any culture that does so

Clerics, priests, and religious leaders have misused the trust placed in them. "The effects of the clerical sex abuse crisis have rippled through the Catholic Church in the United States for decades, and burst into public 20 years ago when the Boston Globe documented a sprawling cover-up of abuse in church settings."[24] Since then, reports and resistance to sex abuse in numerous religious organizations have mounted. In the 696-page report on Illinois' six dioceses, including the Archdiocese of Chicago, it was recorded that since 1950 at least 1,997 children had been abused by clergy members and lay religious brothers. Unlike some states such as California and New York, Illinois does **not** have a "look-back window." A look-back window disregards statutes of limitation and allows survivors of child sex abuse to bring civil claims no matter how long ago the crime happened. Mike McDonnell, a spokesperson for Survivors Network of those Abused by Priests (SNAP), a support network of survivors and advocates who stand by the side of victims, concludes: "This report clearly tells us that no one knew more about abuse, and no one did less about it, than the dioceses themselves."[25] Institutions of any culture can harbor abuses of exploitation and degradation. The church is only one institution that is capable of abuse.

An awareness that the body is a place where God can dwell; this awareness results in actions that respect that holy place

In a Memphis, Tennessee auditorium in 1972, I heard a speaker expound a passage (Ephesians 5:22-33) that talks about submission. This speaker, Bill Gothard, had been recommended by my church. The auditorium was packed with young adults. Bill Gothard interpreted "wives be submissive to your husbands" in this way: If a wife was beaten by her husband, "even to a bloody pulp, she was to submit in the hopes that her husband be won to Christ." That became the day I reexamined the scriptures and my faith.

Susan Hagood Lee stayed for eleven years and thirteen days in an abusive marital relationship. The battering started one month after the ring was safely on her finger. Although she was insulated from family, neighbors, finances, and friends, she had the Bible as a resource. It taught her to pray for those who despitefully used her (Matt. 5:44), to love one who is evil and to offer the second cheek (Matt. 5:38-39). The Bible contained a prohibition of divorce (I Cor. 7:10, 16).[26]

One day her thinking changed. She describes this turning point:

> When I hurt, God hurt; when I was hit, God was hit; when I was bruised, God was bruised; when I could not bear the pain anymore, neither could God. Now this was *not* the God I had hoped for; I was looking for the knight-in-shining-armor God, the God who would gallop in on a white charger, waving a magic wand, and save me! But this rescuer God had been silent; this savior-God was dead. The God I found, the God in agony, the God with me in my pain, became my new God. This God understood my predicament; this God knew what it was to be crucified. This God did *not* want me to suffer; this God wanted me to be happy. But I had to save myself; God would not do it for me. That was the meaning of the

silence. I had to make my own decisions; I was free to make my own decisions; the choice to stay or leave was mine."[27]

A belief that the worth of a person is not based on contour, color, creed, or capabilities

One of the many cases from the autobiography of senior physician Cliff Cleaveland, MD, clearly emphasized the role of the history of a culture. It was difficult for his client, Lena, born in Poland, to undergo some of the treatments prescribed. She put up resistances that were "inappropriate" and "unreasonable." The physician took the time to try to understand the resistance although he did not call it such. Trust was established over time. Then one day, she told him of the camps for prisoners of the third Reich. She and a line of other women who were Jewish were paraded toward a building in the concentration camp. They were required to walk naked. She and others had the fingers of guards stuck up their vaginas as they stood in line. A guard noticed her long blond hair and pulled her out of the line. She was knocked unconscious and raped, but spared. The building at the end of the line was a gas chamber. Only in understanding the dark caverns of her history and culture, could this doctor proceed, with extraordinary care and delicacy, in treatment.[28] "We physicians do not take medical histories so much as we receive them, and this means we must create between our patients and us an unhurried climate of trust and respect."[29]

A commitment to the importance of community in the healing process

In 2017, I was asked to present my sabbatical research on multiple identity politics in relation to personhood, human dignity, and injustice to the Perkins Faculty. My lecture was titled "'So I lost Africa': Personhood, dignity, and multiple identity politics," and it included a case study of Mike whom I had interviewed and followed for years. Raised in Africa until his adolescence, sent to France for education, then to the United States, he displayed what I have termed "cultural dissolution." He described his disorientation, his devastating sense of "rootlessness" and his loss of resources. He said he felt "less than a beggar."

I ended the academic lecture with a personal word to my faculty colleagues. In selecting an example of the role of communities in healing, I selected my own story.[30]

> When our son David died in a terrible car accident (2015), three months before his daughter was born, my husband, our daughter, and I were less than beggars. We had nothing to give. You gave to us: You cleaned our house, took down the Christmas decorations, filled the icebox with food. One of you stood in the driveway upon our return from the funeral in Memphis and welcomed us back with your arms wide open. You gave a Memorial Service. Our Dean told me several times regarding the memorial service: the faculty wanted it. Connie organized, Mark came out of sabbatical and pastored us, the entire choir voluntarily sang, Beka preached of "a sigh too great for words," and all of you shared communion with us—a family of beggars. You taught for me when I could not stand up. You checked on me when I did

begin to teach again. You filled our home with food, and Jim put fresh flowers in my office for weeks when I returned. You took us to quiet places to eat. You listened and you loved as you sighed deeply.

We were beggars with nothing to give. It is an experience of tragedy that I hope you will never understand. This experience of ultimate loss, which to me is the loss of a child, now colors everything I do, all that I write, words that I speak. Like Mike telling his story, I am giving back.

I do not fully understand Mike's story, But I am listening and learning from him and others in pain. For their lives are colored by their experience, and they are giving back. Someday, I am told, the hue of my tragedy will be a different color, but the loss will still be there.

According to sociologist Rodney Clark, there are examples in the early Church of communities surrounding individuals in need, and the communities offering care. "Christianity served as a revitalization movement that arose in response to the misery, chaos, fear, and brutality of life in the urban Greco-Roman world . . . To cities filled with the homeless and impoverished, Christianity offered charity as well as hope. To cities filled with newcomers and strangers, Christianity offered an immediate basis for attachment. To cities filled with orphans and widows, Christianity provided a new and expanded sense of family . . . And to cities faced with epidemics, fire, and earthquakes, Christianity offered effective nursing services."[31]

Conviction about the critical role of the 'holding environment' of the hospital

The common denominators in all lengths of hospitalization and all forms of surgery are still fear of the unknown outcome, discomfort in an unfamiliar environment, a sense of powerlessness and lack of control, and invasion anxiety. Invasion anxiety as a theory has been developed by psychoanalyst Karen Horney in *Feminine Psychology* and, according to Horney, is the counterpart to castration anxiety in men.[32] Many procedures, whether the insertion of tubes, needles or IVs, are invasive to the body. Chemotherapy, radiation, dialysis, and other procedures are intrusive. They may be necessary and life-saving, but they are nevertheless foreign to the natural organism. As physicians of the soul, we create holding environments which help contain anxiety and boundary fear. As one patient's mother described the chaplain: "he took us into the hospital chapel, held our hands, and prayed with us. He had turned an evening of worry and stress into a warm caring circle of shelter." This is a holding environment.

In therapeutic terms, a holding environment is the atmosphere that gives an emotional structure to a person. Patients will need this in the hospital which is an unfamiliar place. Faith is often that which is familiar to a patient. Faith, whatever the tradition, is often the rubric that has given life meaning. By being receptive to the expression of a patient's faith in the hospital, you allow that which is familiar to her or to him to be a part of the hospital experience. Familiar rituals of faith have been shown to also reduce anxiety, lower blood pressure, and decrease stress by producing a relaxation response. Both the rituals of religion and the rituals of medicine are needed in the healing process of the patient. When you, as a physician of the soul, enter the unfamiliar hospital world of IVs, chemotherapy, drips, catheters, and respirators and offer the patient a familiar religious ritual such as Eucharist, anointing with oil or holy water, praying the rosary, the laying on of hands, then the hospital environment takes on a new dimension as a healing community, holding environment, and place of safety.

An understanding of a patient's essential need to feel valued and to be heard

To be a hospital chaplain takes years of training. One of the professional training programs is called Clinical Pastoral Education (CPE). The training is open to all faith denominations and works on something of a mentor system with Certified Clinical Pastoral Educators overseeing the learning. During my CPE residency at Charter Peachford Hospital, Atlanta, (a rehabilitation center for substance abuse) I was called to the bedside of a senior citizen who was in distress. She had already been checked medically, and the opinion was that she was in great emotional pain. I listened—alone—to her detailed recounting of the most traumatic day in her life. Her daughter went to pick up her son (the patient's grandson) from kindergarten. The dismissal process was for the children to wait for the parent/caretaker to circle the cul-de-sac, and then to be led out to the car by a teacher. However, this little boy was so excited to see his mother across the cul-de-sac in a line of cars, that he broke away, ran across the street and was killed by an oncoming car—while his mother watched screaming. For me, the worst pain I could imagine was the loss of a child. Here in slow, graphic detail, I HEARD the agony. I felt the agony. I listened all the way through with deep silence and hidden tears.

An affirmation of both rituals of medicine and rituals in healing

There are rituals in both medicine and religion that occur in a hospital. For example, there is presurgical handwashing, rituals for different types of exams, sterile gloves that meet FDA standards are used in surgery. Larger hospitals will have a staff of chaplains representing different religions. In my own tradition, the use of non-scented holy oil of anointing, the sign of the cross, prayer, and baptism of stillborn or miscarried infants are rituals. There was one nurse, Bonnie, at the Methodist Hospital in Memphis, who developed her own ritual. She always held the hand of a child, teenager, or young adult on the examining table so they would not feel alone or frightened. I remember her strong and comforting hold to this day, and I believe it was the best of both types of rituals.

There is only one piece of literature that I have found written by someone who is both a religious professional and a medical doctor. Franciscan Friar and physician Daniel P. Sulmasy, OFM, MD, affirms both rituals of medicine and healing although he does not practice both in the hospital setting. "I think that they [patients] need both medical and pastoral care, and even though I am among the first to say that ideally these two teams will work closely together for the good of the patient, I am also among the first to say that it is preferable that the boundaries between these two professions be maintained."[33] Not all will agree with this. Hopefully, these two branches of healing, medicine, and spirituality will always join forces.

The rationale behind an oath, whether taking one at medical school graduation or making a vow as one becomes ordained, is to acknowledge publicly and professionally a choice to enter a covenant of care. It is accepting a code of honor that has distinct boundaries and behaviors for the well-being of patients, parishioners, and others we serve.

Misbehavior and misconduct can lurk in the corridors of medicine and religion as we see in contemporary court cases. An oath or credo provides moral parameters to our practices and accountability when these moral borders are breached. The Oath attributed to Hippocrates saw a resurgence of use in medical schools after atrocities committed by medical doctors in the Third Reich were known. Those of us religious professionals are painfully aware of the capitulation of many churches in Germany to the Reich. Our oaths and vows are one way of saying: Never again.

SOULFUL MEDICINE AND SOUL-FILLED MINISTRY

Chaplains communicate a God who protects, who defends, who creates places of safety (Psalms 90 and 91). The work of physicians of the soul and as physicians of the body is to create places of physical and psychological safety as you read in *God's Hotel* by physician Victoria Sweet. A place of safety is a spiritual space. It is a healing place.

Victoria Sweet served as a physician at Laguna Honda Hospital in San Francisco, a hospital or almshouse dedicated to the care of those unable to care for themselves. She came for two months and stayed for twenty years. Sweet learned and practiced "slow medicine" which allowed the amount of time to heal as equivalent to the amount of time it took the illness to develop.[34] She described the healing of one patient,

Terry, as "long, ironic, and miraculous."[35] She goes on to say "Depending on how we label Terry's illness, as transverse myelitis, as a bedsore, as drug abuse, as a poor self-image, or—what I really believe it was—as some deep spiritual wound, two and a half years was just about right."[36] Laguna Honda Hospital, a descendant of the Hotel-Dieu (God's Hotel) in the Middle Ages for the care of the sick and poor, was the last almshouse in the country. It was a hospital with a soul.

"Medicine may be largely a body of knowledge, but healing is a personal skill."[37] For Linda and James Henry, "soul" is an organizing energy in an institution.[38] In comparison to a hospital as a "well-oiled machine," a hospital or clinic with a "soul" is a living, invisible web of interconnectedness.[39] They attribute Hippocrates' ethical standards for medicine as the influence on "the ethical relationship of doctor to patients."[40] This concern inspired the Hippocratic Oath.

Henry and Henry described one of their visits to a medium-sized hospital: "One immediately senses this feeling of soul on entering the hospital and observes it in the delivery of patient care."[41] In other settings, such as Houston Methodist described next, Christ's model of care for the individual is the basis for the ethics in medicine.

HOSPITAL WITH A SOUL

During the January term, I taught a course at Houston Methodist Hospital, which has been ranked by US News & World Report as on the Honor Roll for Best Hospitals in the USA. The Methodist Hospital Care System follows the Methodist Book of Discipline: "We affirm all persons as equally valuable in the sight of God."[42] Under the rubric of the Methodist Church, this hospital strives "to treat everyone as a person of sacred worth and value, created by God."[43] The core values are summarized in an acronym ICARE: Integrity/ Compassion/Accountability/Respect/Excellence. In my first year of teaching there, I often stopped on corners of the labyrinthian hallways to get my bearings. It only took a few seconds for a surgeon with their mask still on or a janitor who knew the halls better than anyone to stop and offer me directions. In terms of kindness, the hospital was a level playing field. I was uplifted by the conscientiousness and dedication of the technology staff, the gift shop attendants, the cafeteria personnel. They endowed the hospital with the essence and enactment of the values of caring. It is a hospital with a soul.

The partnership of physicians of the mind-body-soul is best illustrated to me as I conclude the case of Anne O'Connell. I want to go back to one scene: that of the famous orthopedic surgeon, Dr. F. H. Sims of Mayo Clinic in Rochester, Minnesota and Anne's mother. Anne had undergone five days of testing and had been diagnosed with stage four cancer, an osteogenic sarcoma, a tumor on her right fibula, just below the knee. The leg would have to be amputated above the knee. Her mother approached the doctor and asked about a resection. The doctor agreed to consider it although he had not done it before.

It is this moment, this intervention, of a skillful and famed surgeon from Mayo Clinic coming together with Anne's mother and truly listening, seriously considering this mother's suggestion that has inspired me. Let us not forget that Father Pius and his monks are praying as are many nurses and doctors at Anne's place of employment. For me, this image is what is meant by soulful medicine and soul-filled ministry in partnership. It is the epitome of the Caregiver's Credo.

THE CASE OF ANNE O'CONNELL: PART 3

Reflect on the unknown nature of suffering, how the Hippocratic oath is intended to help, and how the caregiver's credo can be applied to this on-going story.

Anne: "I remember waking up in the recovery room, and Dr. Sims informing me that he was able to save my right leg. He stated that this was the very first time he had performed surgery this way. I was at St. Mary's Hospital for three and a half weeks. My dear mother stayed in Rochester for this time to be with me. She was an example of what deep faith and commitment were."

Two oncologists came into her room twice to present a chemotherapy plan. Anne did not give her consent. On a later day, Dr. Sims came to her room and told her of a panel the doctors had had that morning. They all decided not to start chemotherapy at that time, but if the cancer came back in two and a half years, chemotherapy would be recommended. [A patient with the same cancer had died that morning from his chemotherapy.] She was to have checkups every month for the first year, every two months for the second year, and every three months for the third year. The first year, all checkups were at Mayo. For years two and three, she alternated checkups between Mayo and her home hospital. On one of the home checkups, Anne saw a nurse whom she knew. The nurse told her that the hospital where they had both worked had a mass for Anne before her surgery. She said the chapel was full. This awareness as well as the reports that Dr. Sims at Mayo was continuing to use the resection surgery for other patients meant everything to her.

In October, 1977, Anne was fitted for orthopedic shoes to strengthen her right foot. In the next year, she had a cancerous spot on her left lung. The lung surgery was performed by Dr. Bernautz in 1978 at Mayo Clinic. He removed the small growth. This growth was a loose cell from Jane's first malignancy, osteogenic sarcoma. The growth had traveled from the fibula of her right leg to the lung. Jane has had no recurrence of cancer. She later married and adopted two children.

At a graduation party, a relative of the honoree approached Jane and asked how she was doing. Jane told her medical news. The relative answered: "You are doing okay. And my husband was told from his colon cancer surgery that he would be okay and he died!" Jane got up from the couch, went outside, and wept.

She had just been asked the hardest theological question we religious leaders incur. Why would a benevolent and all-powerful God allow tragedy to happen to a good person? This question or argument is called theodicy, and there are many approaches in an attempt to answer it.[44]

NOTES

1 Howard Thurman, *The Living Wisdom of Howard Thurman: A Visionary for Our Time* (Sounds True: 2010), digital audio.
2 James Cone, *The Spirituals and the Blues*, 2nd revised ed. (Orbis Books, 1992).
3 Cone, *The Spirituals and the Blues*, 104.
4 *Hippocratic Writings*, ed. G. E. R. Lloyd, trans. J. Chadwick and W. N. Mann (London: Penguin Classics, 1978), 50-51. This source explains the word "techne" as art and Greek natural science with rudimentary anatomy and physiology.
5 Victoria Sweet, *God's Hotel: A Doctor, A Hospital, and a Pilgrimage to the Heart of Medicine* (New York: Riverhead, 2012), 79.
6 Sweet, *God's Hotel*, 79.
7 Sweet, *God's Hotel*, 81.
8 This is actually a quote from Dr. Francis Peabody in a speech to the graduating class at Harvard in 1927. God's Hotel, 81.

9 Stephen H. Miles, *The Hippocratic Oath and the Ethics of Medicine* (New York: Oxford University Press, 2004), 2.

10 Walter Bauer, William Arndt, and Wilbur F. Gingrich, *A Greek-English Lexicon of the New Testament and Other Early Christian Literature* (Chicago and London: University of Chicago Press,1957), 585. See also Hayes, Evan, and Stephen Nimis, *Hippocrates' On Airs, Waters and Places and the Hippocratic Oath*, (Oxford, OH: Faenum Publishing, 2013), 107.

11 Miles, *The Hippocratic Oath*, 16.

12 Miles, *The Hippocratic Oath*, 3; repr. of A. A. Pelligrino "Humanism and Ethics in Roman Medicine: Translation and Commentary on a Text of Scribonius Largus," *Lit Med* 7 (1988): 22–38 and J. S. Hamilton, "Scribonius Largus on the medical profession," *Bull Hist Med* 60 (1986): 209–16.

13 Hippocrates, *From The Hippocratic Oath: Text, Translation, and Interpretation,* trans. Ludwig Edelstein (Baltimore: Johns Hopkins Press, 1943), 3–63. Also, found in translation from Greek by Ludwig Edelstein. *Ancient Medicine: Selected Papers of Ludwig Edelstein,* eds. Owsei Temkin and C. Lilian Temkin (Baltimore & London: Johns Hopkins Press, 1967), 6.

14 Credo is the Latin for "I believe." A credo can be in the form of a creed such as the Nicene Creed or it can be a statement of one's set of principles or a belief system. In this book, I am using the latter meaning.

15 Marie Fortune, *Is Nothing Sacred? When Sex Invades the Pastoral Relationship* (San Francisco: Harper, 1992)

16 G.E.T. Lord, introduction to *Hippocratic Writings* (London: Penguin Books, 1978), 59–60.

17 William Bynum, *The History of Medicine: A Very Short Introduction* (Oxford University Press, 2008), 5

18 Bynum, *The History of Medicine,* 7.

19 This list is an expanded version from the one found in Stevenson-Moessner, Jeanne, preface to *Women Out of Order: Risking Change and Creating Care in a Multicultural World,* eds. Jeanne Stevenson-Moessner and Bishop Teresa Snorton, (Minneapolis: Fortress Press, 2000), 2.

20 Eduardo Duran, *Healing the Soul Wound: Trauma Informed Counseling for Indigenous Communities,* 2nd ed (New York: Teachers College Press, Columbia University, 2019), 13.

21 Eduardo Duran, "Healing with Dignity: Spiritual/Pastoral Care in Native America" conference at Perkins School of Theology, SMU, plenary address, March 30, 2023.

22 Rebecca Skloot, *The Immortal Life of Henrietta Lacks* (New York: Random House, 2010).

23 Maria Cheng, "Lawsuits: Canada's Indigenous Women still forcibly sterilized," *Telegraph Herald*, July 23, 2023, p.8C.

24 Ruth Graham, "Sex Abuse in the Catholic Church: Over 1,900 Minors Abused in Illinois, State Says", *The New York Times,* May 23, 2023. https://www.nytimes.com/2023/05/23/us/illinois-catholic-sex-abuse.html

25 Graham, "Sex Abuse in the Catholic Church".

26 Susan Lee Hagood, "Witness to Christ, Witness to Pain: One Women's Journey Through Wife Battering," in *Sermons Seldom Heard: Women Proclaim Their Lives,* ed. Annie Lally Milhaven (New York: Crossroad Press, 1991), 11–22.

27 Hagood, "Witness to Christ," 15.

28 Cleaveland, *Sacred Space*, 140–45.

29 Cleaveland, *Sacred Space*, 145.

30 Our son's school (Nativity Catholic School in Dubuque), my home community in Memphis, Wesleyan Hills UMC, and our Dallas church (First Presbyterian) formed similar healing, holding environments for us.

31 Rodney Stark, *The Rise of Christianity* (Princeton University Press, 1996), 161.

32 Karen Horney, *Feminine Psychology* (New York: W.W.Norton, 1967), 69.

33 Sulmsy, Daniel P., O.F.M., M.D., *The Healer's Calling: A Spirituality for Physicians and Other Health Care Professionals, (*New York: Paulist Press, *1997),* 67–68.

34 Sweet, *God's Hotel*, 98.

35 Sweet, *God's Hotel*, 98.

36 Sweet, *God's Hotel*, 98.

37 Ray Porter, in Linda Gambee Henry and James Douglas Henry, *Reclaiming Soul in Health Care: Practical Strategies for Revitalizing Providers of Care* (Chicago: American Hospital Association Press, 1999), 43.

38 Henry and Henry, *Reclaiming Soul*, 27.

39 Henry and Henry, *Reclaiming Soul*, 38.

40 Henry and Henry, *Reclaiming Soul*, 39.

41 Henry and Henry, *Reclaiming Soul*, 29.

42 *Book of Discipline of the United Methodist Church* (Nashville: The United Methodist Publishing House, 2016), 119.

43 *Living Houston Methodist Values: A Handbook for Employees/2016.* The quote is on page 1 and the ICARE values listed on page18.

44 Jeffrey Zurheide, *When Faith is Tested: Pastoral Responses to Suffering and Tragic Death* (Minneapolis: Fortress Press, 1997). Zurheide offers typical answers to the question: Why would a good and omnipotent God allow this tragedy to happen? Common responses are God is teaching you something; God is testing you; God is training you for something; God is punishing you; It is God's will. In the end, Zurheide comes out with the belief: "theodicy is a mystery; suffering is at its core mystery; God is mystery." (p.73) "Make your lips form the words: I don't know". (p.75) "In addition to our presence, humility, and tears, we can offer the perspective—in our own words—God will not leave you alone. God is with you."

FOUR

Dis-eases of the Soul

THE SIN-SICK SOUL

John Chrysostom viewed the priest as a doctor of the soul. Chrysostom utilized medical imagery through-out all of his writings. He even conceived "of his school—the church—as a medical clinic (*iatreion*)[1] and, as a philosopher-teacher-priest, the guidance and healing of sick souls as fundamental to his job description."[2] Chrysostom believed that sin caused sickness. The sicknesses of the soul Chrysostom strove to cure as physician, "are not metaphoric or analogous, but literal and genuine."[3] In his homilies on Romans, John Chrysostom lists these dis-eases of the soul: ungodliness/unrighteousness (Rom 1:18), vile affections (Rom 1: 24, 26), reprobation (Rom 1:28) and deceit which is likened to the poison of asps under the lips.[4] This is why the diseases necessitate the cutting with the knife—to remove the venom, the sepsis. The more profuse the infection, the sharper the knife. In Chrysostom's homilies on Galatians and Ephesians, the dis-eases continue: walking unworthy of the vocation wherewith you are called (Eph IV: 1-3), walking in the vanity of the mind (Eph IV: 17), being alienated from the life of God, lying (Eph IV:25-30), speaking evil with malice (Eph IV: 31, 32), being an idolater (Eph V:5-14). The lists, which continue in Galatians, include frustrating the grace of God (Gal II.21).[5]

Theology works best in the interstices or intersections of church history, systematics, Bible, ethics, specialized anthropological studies, pastoral theology, practical theology, and art.[6] A theology of healing works best when there is a connection among theologians, medical doctors, medical personnel, psychiatrists, psychologists, therapists, and physicians of the soul. The connection between sin and sickness was made by John Chrysostom and other church fathers. A vice is a sin. The opposite of a vice is a virtue. Whoever has control of naming the vices, can name the virtues. Whoever can name the virtues has power to assess the human condition. The power is in the naming. Those who categorized the seven deadly sins were in an influential position. However, the categorization of the seven deadly sins or the heptad is not sufficient for all people today.[7]

The objective of this chapter is to revisit the categorization and depiction of the "seven deadly sins," to reenvision them, and to offer instead a triad of evil. In doing so, I will later offer a trinity of virtues. Examining vices and virtues offers a commentary on the condition of a society or that of humankind. Is the society riddled with vices? Do virtues (moral, intellectual, social) balance or outweigh the vices? With these questions in mind, physicians of souls can both listen more effectively and speak more accurately into the situation of humankind.

DIS-EASES OF THE SOUL

Many of John Chrysostom's examples of healing attribute the sickness to the sufferer's sin or lack of virtue. However, in the examples of Christ healing, not all of the physical illnesses were caused by personal or internal sin. In the two following examples, the sin came from external or outside forces, one familial and the other political. The medical profession prefers the use of the unhyphenated word *disease*. The cause could be idiopathic or indicative of an unknown cause. The cause could be known: genetic, environmental, an imbalance in the body's chemistry, bacteria, viruses, fungi. parasites, protozoa, helminths (worms). In the following example, the hyphenated word, *dis-ease*, will be used to indicate spiritual septicity, a discomfort, an imbalance, a pain,or a wounding of the soul. Chrysostom was focused on a soul at ease with it Creator. Therefore, any sin or violence to the soul would put the soul into a state of disequilibrium or dis-ease. The following case will feature Marge who suffered from an anxiety disorder which put her perpetually in a state of dis-ease. As this case unfolds, you will see the rationale and reality of this condition. Violence at an early age had wounded her soul.

Marge was described to me as "stuck in therapy" and in need of relaxation/meditative exercises. Marge, a forty-five-year-old-female, was referred to me by the clinical psychologist who served as Director of the Gannon Center for Community Mental Health in Dubuque, Iowa. He asked me to work with Marge as a supplement to his weekly counseling sessions with her. He had been treating Marge for an anxiety disorder and saw little progress.

I tried various techniques. Marge was unable to relax or meditate with any of the conventional methods because of recurring alarming and intrusive thoughts when she was physically inactive.

As our weeks together unfolded, Marge let me know gradually that she had been seriously abused as a child. The abuse occurred in various parts of her childhood home, most notably the dank and unlit basement where she was locked in a cellar for long periods. I once suggested that we imagine we were sitting on a beach looking at the ocean and relaxing together. Marge was afraid something would come from behind and grab her or that the ocean itself would drag her away into the deep. We tried this exercise by imagining other locations like a mountain side, but the same fears arose. I felt stuck.

I had been well-trained not to reveal much if anything about myself. In this Center for Community Mental Health, open to all faith traditions or lack thereof, we were not to mention religious affiliation lest it be taken as proselytizing. In order to form a beginning level of trust, I offered to answer two questions about myself. I knew the choices Marge made in forming and selecting the questions would give me significant leads on her "being stuck" in therapy. Marge asked:

1. Do you know what it is like to have your heart broken? Yes.
2. Do you have children? Yes.

A relationship of trust was forming, I believe, as I offered a glimpse of my vulnerability.

And this is when things began to change. I won the raffle at the neighborhood Catholic church for the big prize. The coveted raffle prize was a magnificently, tastefully, and lovingly decorated doll's house (see color insert). The women's church guild had fashioned it, and each room had such warmth, color, and cozy detail.

I brought this house into therapy. It was something Marge had never seen before, hence, there were no immediate negative associations. It was completely open in the back. The bedroom had a hole in the floor under the bed so that no one could be trapped in that room. There was no attic, and especially no basement. Marge and I spent a lot of time through our imagination in that living room. We pretended to order out and imagined a catering service delivering luscious food to the front door. We had high tea with pastries. We had margaritas. We laughed, we talked, and we relaxed in a safe environment—devoid of any abusive memories.

My inclination to develop this technique, which in psychology is called a safe space, stems from my spirituality and my research on women's development. The technique I developed is *imaginative relocation*. The fact that there was an actual house before us helped us springboard into the imaginative exercise. Although I was never to mention my faith affiliation, my concept of safety stems from my understanding of a God who protects, who defends, who creates places of safety.[8] My awareness of women's development in a culture that is often harmful or stifling to women prompted me to create a safe place for relaxation and meditation. Conservative estimates show that "rape is committed against one out of four women in the United States; one third of female children and adolescents under the age of eighteen experience significant sexual abuse; and violence occurs in one-third of U.S. families."[9] This will also be the work of physicians of the soul and physicians of the mind: to create places of physical and psychological safety. A place of safety can be a spiritual space, a sanctuary of healing.

The previous failed attempts to help Marge feel safe and secure showed us she was suffering from dis-ease in her soul. This dis-ease was an anxiety disorder that was brought on by Adverse Childhood Experiences (ACE). Trauma was inflicted on her in her childhood home.

Abusive parents infected her childhood development so that mistrust won out over trust.[10] It could also be that she was suffering from Posttraumatic Stress Disorder (PTSD).[11] It was the clinical psychologist's role to listen, discern, diagnose, treat, and hopefully cure. My assigned role was to create a safe place where she could relax and begin to trust that therapeutic environment. Marge did not know that I was also a minister. I did not say that the parents had sinned against her; that their traumatization of her was a sin. I did say that nothing she had done was wrong. That what her parents had done was terribly wrong.

It was an honor to be asked by the Director of the Gannon Center to use my training as a minister and pastoral counselor to help Marge. I did not cure, nor heal, Marge. That was not my assignment. However, I did sense the depth of the childhood trauma of her soul and was able to create a safe and eventually enjoyable place. We sat together in a space I would call sacred.

THE EYES OF EVIL

The role of the church is to protect us from evil that is all around us, including the evil within us. The Swiss artist Stefan à Wengen produced forty-nine *Geister-Porträten* (ghost portraits) by taking faces of ordinary people and putting the eyes of evil people in their faces. Wengen chose ordinary people and replaced their innocence with the "eyes of evil." These eyes came from dictators, tyrants, and fundamentalists like Adolf Hitler, Stalin, and Khomeini.[12] "Existing in these portraits are eyes—like mirrors to the soul—from so-called icons of fundamentalism, dictators, and tyrants of ancient and modern history."[13] Wengen wanted to remind us that humans, ordinary humans, are filled with evil as well.

Each morning while a visiting professor at the University of Luzern, I could hear from my room in the Priesterseminar St. Beat the sounds of the Lord's prayer: "And lead us not into Temptation, but deliver us from evil."[14] I looked out of the windows in the refectory at breakfast, and I saw each day the gargoyles of the neighboring St. Leodegar Church. The gargoyles surrounded the church also to protect the church itself from evil all around us.

I was invited to sit in on the research of Professor Dr. Markus Ries and his assistant Valentin Beck, Dr. Markus Furrur (PHZ Luzern), Prof. Stephanie Klein, and others from the Diocese of Luzern and the University Luzern. Their research had been commissioned by the Roman Catholic Church and civil authorities in Kanton Luzern. This research collaboration was bold and courageous and a model of the church and theologians working to name evil. The research attempts to see through the eyes of victims/survivors of child sexual abuse in Catholic orphanages in the diocese of Luzern. Sadly, the abuses had been inflicted by nuns and priests. When abuse occurs within specific religious settings, the negative aspects of certain religious symbols and the consequences of certain Christian virtues and values must be examined and re-examined.

For example, even suffering sexual assault can be sanctified and uplifted by the church. According to her authorized biographers, Maria Goretti at age eleven refused to be raped by a relative. She fought back, was stabbed fourteen times, and died in a hospital. The church glorified her suffering because she fought to be a virgin. She died a virgin. Before she died, she forgave the assailant. According to the church authorities, her suffering was known by God before it happened. Through her suffering she received holiness. Thus, according to her biographers and their interpretation, sexual assault can be a blessing in disguise. Maria Goretti became a saint in 1950. She was used as a model for Catholic youth in a papal address by Pope John Paul in 1980. Whoever has control of naming the vices, can name the virtues.

Five of the virtues in Maria's case were as follows: "(1) the value of suffering; (2) the virtue of forgiveness; (3) the [virtue] of remaining sexually pure (especially for little girls); (4) the [virtue] of redemption; and, most important, (5) the value that is placed on their obedience to authority figures."[15] Sheila Redmond then goes on to discuss these five virtues or points through the "eyes" of the Christian child who has been sexually assaulted by someone she or he knows. It is time to re-examine who controls the naming of virtues.

THE SEVEN DEADLY SINS

The history of the classification of the deadly sins is important because only certain men had the power of naming. The introduction of the term "deadly sins" has been traced to the "Testament of Reuben," in the pseudepigraphal Testaments of the Twelve Patriarchs, the Sons of Jacob the Patriarch (109–106 BCE). In this Testament of Reuben, seven spirits of deceit are named: promiscuity, insatiability, strife, flattery, arrogance, lying, and injustice.[16] The idea of a group of deadly sins comes in waves and in subsequent writings up to the thirteenth century. The next grouping of deadly sins comes later in the practical guides of Evagrius Ponticus (346–399 CE); Evagrius Ponticus was one of the desert fathers in the early church and a monastic theologian. Evagrius listed eight demons or thoughts that plagued monks; it is crucial to note that his list was written for ascetic and desert anchorites. The demons or vices were as follows: gluttony, impurity, avarice, sadness, anger, sloth, vainglory, and pride. They were in no systematic order.

Traditionally, the seven deadly sins were listed as following:[17] pride, envy, wrath(anger), sloth, avarice, gluttony, and lust. Whereas pride was often depicted as the root sin for theologians at this time, for Chrysostom it was the worship of Mammon—a biblical term for possessions and riches. "Let us then, bearing in mind all these things, flee the incurable disease; let us heal the wounds it has made, and withdraw ourselves from such a pest."[18] Mammon is also a wealth of power accumulated by any means. Chrysostom uses King Herod as an example. Herod's monopoly of power was threatened by a child for whom the Magi searched. Herod is dis-eased by the cancer of anger. He directs his anger to children under the age of two. This became the slaughter of the innocents in Bethlehem.

Many contemporaries of John Chrysostom were influenced by Evagrius, including Chrysostom's biographer, Palladius, a student of Evagrius. Whereas Evagrius was a follower of Origen,[19] Evagrius had a follower in John Cassian. John Cassian (fourth to fifth century CE) transmitted the list of vices to the Latin monastic tradition and to the Western church. Cassian described the monk as an athlete for Christ, battling these sins. Augustine (fourth to fifth century CE) embellished the list of vices. Gregory the Great (sixth century CE) shortened the list to seven vices by subsuming sloth under sadness, adding envy as a vice, and separating pride as the root. Gregory the Great as well as Cassian

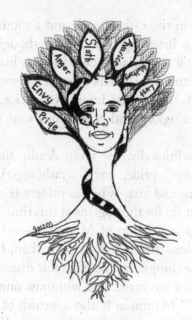

The seven deadly sins. Drawing by Jean Stevenson Moessner.

arranged the sins on a continuum from carnal vices to spiritual ones, thus gluttony was at one end and pride at the other. Gregory called pride "the mother and Queen of all vices." Gregory gave the seven vices authoritative status: "scholastic theologians systematized [them] in the 13th century, and [they] appeared extensively in penitential and preaching manuals after the Fourth Lateran Council (1215)."[20] Thomas Aquinas was one of the 13th century theologians who systematized the heptad or seven vices and virtues. The "seven deadly sins" had been classified out of masculine experience. Evagrius concluded that women and bishops constituted the greatest temptation to monks, and both [women and bishops] should be avoided whenever possible! There is definitely a bias at play. The seven deadly sins became, to some, like a viper's poison to the soul.

There is not a list in the Bible that explicitly names the seven deadly sins, although scattered biblical references to sin have influenced the list. The phrase "seven deadly sins" has been classified out of masculine experience. In 1960, a theologian named Valerie Saiving Goldstein upset the traditional construct or classification of "the seven deadly sins" with the publication of her article, "The Human Situation: A Feminine View".[21] Arguing that theological doctrines were primarily constructed on the basis of masculine experience, Valerie Saiving Goldstein went on to contest the sin of pride from the basis of feminine experience. For women, rather than pride, the vice was "underdevelopment or negation of the self."[22] This can also be expressed as *selflessness*. In Valerie Saiving's words:

> The specifically feminine forms of sin have a quality which can never be encompassed by such terms as "pride" or "will-to-power." They are better suggested by such terms as triviality, distractibility, and diffuseness; lack of an organizing center or focus; dependence on others for one's own self-definition; tolerance at the expense of standards of excellence; inability to respect the boundaries of privacy; sentimentality, gossipy sociability, and mistrust of reason—in short, underdevelopment or negation of the self.[23]

Valerie Saiving attributed these feminine forms of temptations and sins to the basic feminine character structure which is formed by anatomy, socialization, and the capacity for surrendering individual concerns to serve the immediate needs of others. Her goal was to "awaken theologians" to seeing the feminine experience more accurately.[24] For example, a sin like wrath and its corresponding virtue (meekness, patience) can be misconstrued to foster submission in women that has unhealthy if not deadly consequences. Jesus modeled wrath when moneychangers defiled the temple. What kind of wrath is a sin? Is the absence of justified and healthy anger also a sin? This is one example of the work that lies ahead for physicians of the soul.

The African-American experience of pride is also not represented by the classical depiction. Oxford University Press has published a series on the seven deadly sins. Michael Eric Dyson, Professor of Religious Studies and Africana Studies at the University of Pennsylvania chose to write the volume on pride: "I also chose the most deadly of the seven sins because I wanted to deepen my engagement with pride, not only as a philosophical and religious idea but especially as a racial and national force."[25] Michael Eric Dyson refers to Aristotle's notion of "proper pride" and relates it to his pride of race as an African American. He summarizes: "despite the thematic consistency across diverse Christian communities—pride is viewed as the basic sin in RC parishes as well as in black Baptist churches—just what pride looks like and how it is best addressed is colored by the social and political contexts that shape faith and theology."[26] Although all of the Oxford University Press volumes bear creative insights such as Dyson's, the rubric for the volumes are the traditional seven deadly sins. It is time to reimagine and reinterpret the rubric of the sins with a fresh, realistic interpretation for our day.

In *The Canterbury Tales* of Geoffrey Chaucer, written at the end of the fourteenth century, it was the wise parson who interpreted the seven capital (deadly) sins into the culture of his day:[27] "We are asked to consider the extravagance of our clothing, the greediness of landlords, the richness of our food, the deceit of merchants, the raising of our children, the backbiting of gossips, and much more in the same vein—all of them examples from our ordinary behavior, no less relevant now than six hundred years ago."[28] This type of interpretation and application is necessary for the twenty-first century. Noteworthy is the fact that the country parson, a poor but holy Protestant minister of a parish, gives of his own stipend to his parishioners in need. He models the honest reexamination of the meaning of the seven vices.

TOWER OF BABEL: INDUSTRY AS VICE

Let us now see how a vice or virtue can be reenvisioned. Sloth or lack of industry is one of the classic "Seven Deadly Sins." Today, we might label a slothful person as a slacker, an idler, one who avoids work or effort. The French artist Jacques Callot illustrated sloth as an inactive woman who appeared to be in contemplation or meditation. The following case study titled "Tower of Babel" attempts to show that industry, when consisting of meaningless or manipulative activity, can in itself be a vice.

Sharon's mother taught her that the church was a safe haven and a place of authority. The church was the "center of everything." The option to stay home from church on a Sunday morning never presented itself in her childhood in a small Nebraska town (in the midwestern part of the USA). Sharon's aunt picked her up on Wednesday nights for Bible study and took her to play her guitar at the local nursing home. Sharon described the church as her "plumb line" or her measure of all that was good.

Sharon followed a call into ministry and completed her theological training. She and her husband, Tim, had two children. When Tim died of a brain tumor, Sharon was left at forty-three years of age with two children in college. Sharon expected the church would continue to give her the grace and the strength she needed.

Sharon was appointed by the United Methodist Church (UMC) to a small city church with serious financial debts. As their new pastor, she was responsible to improve the financial shortfall. She managed to get the church on solid financial footing and pay apportionments to the UMC. There was no funding for new buildings. Sharon endured gender discrimination and lack of support as a female. One overbearing bishop reprimanded Sharon and told her God would not say "well done, good and faithful servant" upon her entrance into God's full presence in heaven. Biting her lip, she replied: "Yes, God will, if I am faithful." The bishop threatened to suspend her if she ever told of their encounter. The bishop abused his power.

She was reassigned to a rural church which resulted in an annual salary reduction of $14,000. Sharon named the cardinal sin in many institutional churches today and in many leaders of the churches as "the Tower of Babel" or the building of a personal kingdom. This personal kingdom requires that a pastor have a large and dedicated following, a loyal populace with money, and devotees. She maintains: "It is not the numbers, rather it is the one or two persons who find their way to Christ." She believes there is a greed for power in the church. Man-made industry can erect a "tower of Babel" to reach to heaven. This misplaced industry is a vice as injurious as the traditional understanding of sloth (Socordia).

Sharon continues to serve a small church in rural Nebraska. Her church is growing, in a heightened sense of community, in outreach to the community, in its music ministry, in deepening spirituality among its members, and in numbers.[29]

A TRINITY OF VIRTUE, A TRIAD OF VICE

The traditional formulation of seven deadly sins, the heptad, reflects the masculine experience that limits the interpretation and application of sins. It is time to venture into new images. There is no foundation for the construct of a heptad or seven deadly vices in either the Hebrew Bible or the New Testament. Rather there is a trinity of virtue: Love of self, love of God, love of neighbor[30]; on these three loves, hang all the law and prophets according to three writers, Matthew, Mark, and Luke. The New Testament books that bear the names of the writers are called the synoptic Gospels because of similar stories and sequences. The words attributed to Christ in Matthew 22:34-40, Mark 12:28-34, and Luke 10:25-37 use Leviticus 19:18 and Deuteronomy 6:5 as prequel.

A lawyer tries to trick Jesus into answering the question: What must I do to gain eternal life? Jesus referred him to the law: "Love God with all your heart, mind, and soul, and your neighbor as yourself." Following the lawyer's question and Jesus's answer, there is the parable of the Good Samaritan. A man traveled from Jerusalem to Jericho and was stripped and beaten by robbers. The poor sojourner was left for half-dead. A priest passed by as did a Levite. But the least likely person to stop, a Samaritan, had pity or compassion on the beaten traveler and stopped to help. The Samaritan bandaged the wounds, poured water and oil on them. The

Samaritan enlisted the aid of an animal to transport the wounded to an inn. Then the Samaritan gave the innkeeper money to care for the wounded. The Samaritan spent a refreshing night in the inn.

The Samaritan finished her/his journey. The Samaritan left the wounded with the innkeeper, finished his journey, and followed up with aftercare. The Samaritan not only paid the innkeeper; the Samaritan said anything remaining as debt would be repaid upon the return visit. The Samaritan managed to care for the wounded, while finishing the journey. By finishing her journey, the Samaritan exhibited self-care and love of self. By delegating the responsibilities in caring and relying on other professionals (i.e. the innkeeper), the Samaritan avoided compassion fatigue. For many physicians of the soul and perhaps those in other helping professionals, we have missed the permission, if not command, to love ourselves. We hesitate to delegate responsibilities and to collaborate in our healing professions.

We will need fresh theological images such as that of loving self as well as God and others. Images are absorbed; concepts are learned.[31] According to the late Nelle Morton, we can change concepts through education and rational thinking. However, to change an image, it must be shattered. That makes way for a new image to form in the soul. I found such an image while climbing the precarious and endless scaffolding to the dome of the Samford University Hodges Chapel: the depiction of the Holy Trinity.[32] I was able to purchase the cartoon[33] of this trinity later (see color insert).

The antitheses of these three virtues comprise and cover the list of more than the classical seven deadly sins. A triad of vice could be hatred, theft, the underdevelopment or negation of the self. For example, love of God is negated by hatred of many hues; love of neighbor

PHYSICIAN OF SOULS

is extinguished when there is hording of resources; love of self is impossible when there is degradation or deprivation of the self. Contemporary paintings and other art forms can shatter old images as we find new ways to express both the virtues and the vices, the good and the evil, judgment and grace.

The work of theologians can be inspired by the artistic and contemporary rendition of deadly sins as portrayed in the work of artist Jacques Richard Chery from Haiti. This painting hangs in the administration building of the Latin American Biblical University in San Jose, Costa Rica. It was first explained to me as glimpses of "the invisible Christ" because Christ (in red attire) appears in some form in each segment. Christ is moving among the vices: dislocation, violence, oppression, homelessness, exclusion, hunger, unemployment, violation of human rights, idolatry. The actual title of the art is the Meseror hunger cloth from Haiti- The Tree of Life 1982.

The work as physicians of the soul can be inspired by artists creating new images, listening, and renaming sins. The Kunstmuseum (art museum) in Luzern featured Katerina Seda from the Czech Republic. Based on a Czech proverb, her project was titled: "Talk to the sky because the ground isn't [ain't] listening." If the ground doesn't listen, hopefully we theologians and pastors can.

Katerina Seda's project started when she observed the despair of her grandmother, Jana. Her grandmother retired after 33 years as a tools stock manager in a hardware store. She memorized over 650 types of goods and their prices. When she retired, the grandmother decided she would do nothing. She stopped cooking, cleaning, and shopping, and spent all of her time in front of the television. Her answer to questions was: "It doesn't matter." ["Es ist mir egal."] Katerina Seda helped her grandmother literally draw her way out of this meaninglessness of despair. Surely the belief that my life or your life or Jana Seda's life doesn't matter is evil. There is power is in the naming.

A feminist theology of sin, according to Joy Ann McDougall, must "specify the particular forms of blockage or blindness to which women fall prey. In what concrete ways do women both refuse and are themselves refused God's good gifts of grace? Here both feminist theorists and theologians play a critical part in exposing those gender specific forces that obstruct women's self-development and social flourishing."[34]

In his book, *Seven Deadly Sins: A Very Partial List*, Aviad Kleinberg opens with this: "Christianity is founded on sin. Not that its founders were sinners; on the contrary, they seem to be upright men. But sin is the foundation of the Christian worldview. The Christian is first and foremost a sinner, and Christianity constitutes above all a remedy for sin."[35] If this perception is anywhere near true, we have our work before us as theologians. For the sins of today need renaming. The renaming includes sins such as ethnic cleansing, holocausts, devastation of Mother Earth, human rights violations, terror, bullying, and all manner of violence.[36] Above all we must remember: "For He [Christ] came as a Physician, not as a Judge."[37]

We as physicians of the soul are in a powerful position. Although we may not be artists like Stefan à Wengen or Katerina Seda, we are the verbal artists who can translate both virtue and vice for a new age. To understand dis-eases of the soul, an examination of the history of the "seven deadly sins," a theological construct that has dominated the church's understanding and nomenclature of evil, is an important place to start. However, it is now time to update our advances in understanding dis-eases of the soul. There are medical manuals and databases for physicians of the body, but they need constant revisions

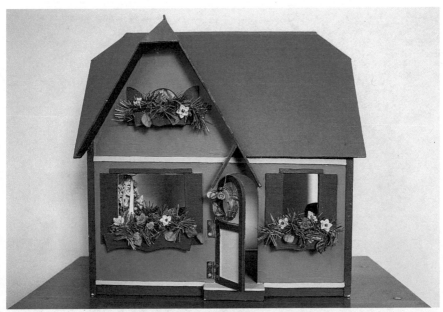

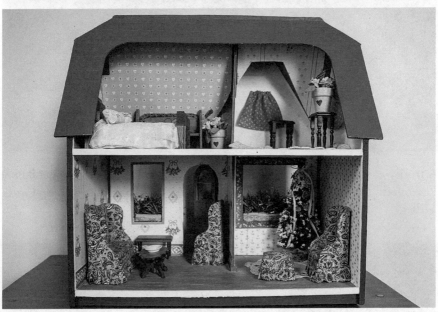

Sitting room of doll's house used as safe space in therapy. No basement, open doors and windows, no attic, open space under the bed, no back wall. Made lovingly by the Women's Auxiliary at Nativity School and Church. Alta Vista Street, Dubuque, Iowa. Photographer: Gwen Gross Miller.

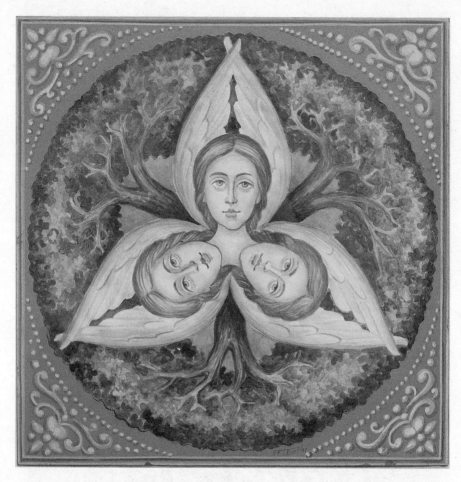

A trinity of virtues representing the three loves: love of God, love of neighbor, love of self. Artist: Petru Botezatu from Romania. Photographer: Gwen Gross Miller.

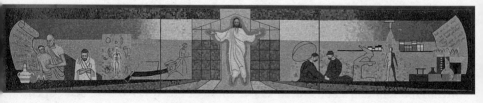

Extending Arms of Christ Mural. Artist: Bruce Hayes.

as advances are made in medicine.[38] There is a manual for physicians of the mind, psychologists, and mental health workers which is now in a fifth edition.[39] Physicians of the soul are informed by the holy scriptures of respective faith traditions. We can be the brokers of a refurbished and revitalized vocabulary. It is time to appraise, for example, the trinity of virtues and the triad of vices. We can be translators of revised theological concepts and spiritual insights for healing of the wounds of the soul.

NOTES

1 Wendy Mayer, "John Chrysostom: Moral Philosopher and Physician of the Soul," in *John Chrysostom Past, Present, Future*, eds. Doru Costache and Mario Baghos (Sydney, AIOCS Press, 2017), 214-15.

2 Mayer, "John Chrysostom," 214.

3 Mayer, "John Chrysostom," 214.

4 Library of the Fathers of the Holy Catholic Church, S. *Chrysostom's Homilies on Romans*, vol. 7, (Oxford: John Henry Parker, 1841).

5 Library of the Fathers of the Holy Catholic Church, S. *Chrysostom's Homilies on Galatians and Ephesians*, vol. 5, ed. Rev. W. J. Copeland (Oxford: John Henry Parker, 1840).

6 Jeanne Stevenson-Moessner, *Prelude to Practical Theology: Variations on Theory and Practice* (Nashville: Abingdon Press, 2008), 1. In this book, I have used the theme of practical theology as the music of theological inquiry which gives practical theologians opportunity to create beyond the formal disciplines of their training. We play in concert with other disciplines such as art, church history, ethics.)

7 The Christian ascetic Evagrius Ponticus, who created the list of seven, later added "sloth" as the eighth deadly sin.

8 Psalms 90, 91

9 Jean Baker Miller, *Toward a New Psychology of Women* (Boston: Beacon Press, 1976), 53, in *In Her Own Time: Women and Developmental Issues in Pastoral Care*, ed. Jeanne Stevenson-Moessner (Minneapolis, Fortress Press, 2000), 3.

10 Erik Erikson developed psychosocial stages of development. His first stage was trust versus mistrust which is the psychological challenge of a child from birth to 18 months. Then, autonomy versus shame and doubt is the challenge to a child 18 months to three years. There are eight stages in this epigenetic progression, and each stage has a major resolution or conflict to resolve. See *Childhood and Society*, 2nd ed. (New York: Norton, 1993).

11 PTSD is a persistent condition of stress (mental and emotional) that follows a trauma or injury. One common symptom is intrusive thoughts or images such as being grabbed from behind in Marge's case. Being in an enclosed space could have also brought back memories.

12 Wengen called the eyes "Augen des Bösen."

13 Wengen "Vorlagen zu diesen Porträts sind Augen—gewissermassen als Spiegel der Seele—von sogenannten Icons von Fundamentalisten, Diktatoren und Tyrannen der älteren und jüngeren Geschichte."

14 Matthew 6:9-13 and in Luke 11:1-4 in the New Testament.
    The nuns faithfully prayed daily: Vater Unser. "Und fuhre uns nicht in Versuchung, sondern erloese uns von dem Boesen (Uebel)."

15 Sheila A. Redmond, "Christian 'Virtues' and Recovery from Child Sexual Abuse," in *Christianity, Patriarchy, and Abuse: A Feminist Critique*, eds. Joanne Carlson Brown and Carole R. Bohn (New York: Pilgrim Press, 1989), 74.

16 H. C. Kee, "Testaments of the Twelve Patriarchs (Second Century B.C.)" in *The Old Testament Pseudepigrapha: Apocalyptic Literature & Testaments*, ed. James Charlesworth (Garden City: Doubleday, 1983), 782–83. The seven spirits of error arise from Reuben's penitence over his rape of Bilhah.

17 The seven corresponding virtues are as follows: humility, kindness, patience, diligence, liberality, abstinence, chastity.

18 Matt 2:16; Chrysostom, "Homily IX," 170

19 It has been noted that this was a conflictual relationship.

20 Rebecca Konyndyk DeYoung, "The Seven Deadly Sins," in vol. 5 (Si-Z) *Encyclopedia Christianity* (Grand Rapids: Eerdmans, 2008), 25.

21 Valerie Saiving Goldstein, "The Human Situation: A Feminine View," *Journal of Religion*, 40 (1960):100-112.

22 Saiving Goldstein, "The Human Situation", 109.

23 Saiving Goldstein, "The Human Situation," 109.

24 Saiving Goldstein, "The Human Situation," 109.

25 Michael Eric Dyson, preface to *Pride* (New York: Oxford University Press, 2006). "The notion of pride is perhaps even more ethically useful to humans the world over now that we are living again through ethnic cleansings, holocausts, civil rights revolutions, famines, human rights struggles, wars, and all manner of terror." P.6.

26 Dyson, *Pride*, 13.

27 Henry Fairlie, *The Seven Deadly Sins Today* (Washington: New Republic Books, 1978), 13.

28 Fairlie, *The Seven Deadly Sins Today*, 13.

29 Sharon's steadfast service to the church represents the unsullied nature of industry as a virtue. The search for power, money and devotees is a tainted and contaminated substitute for industry which now becomes a vice. An expanded description can be found in *The Elephant in the Church: What You Don't See Can Kill Your Ministry*, Jeanne Stevenson-Moessner and Mary Lynn Dell, MD, (Nashville: Abingdon Press, 2013) 33–43.

30 Jeanne Stevenson-Moessner, "A New Pastoral Paradigm and Practice," in *Women in Travail and Transition: A New Pastoral Care,* eds. Maxine Glaz and Jeanne Stevenson-Moessner (Minneapolis: Fortress Press, 1991), 200–204.

31 Nelle Morton, *The Journey is Home* (Boston: Beacon Press, 1985), 31

32 The depiction of the Holy Trinity is beside Athanasius, bishop of Alexandria, Egypt. Artist: Petru Botezatu.

33 A full-scale initial painting in preparation for the final rendition.

34 Joy Ann McDougall, "Sin—No More? A Feminist Re-Visioning of a Christian Theology of Sin," in *Anglican Theological Review*, 88 (Spring 2006): 215–35.

35 Aviad Kleinberg, *7 Deadly Sins: A Very Partial List* (Cambridge: Harvard University Press, 2008), 10.

36 Dyson, preface to *Pride,* 6.

37 Matt 1:1; Chrysostom, Homily III, 62.

38 For example: Robert E. Porter, *Merck Manual of Diagnosis and Therapy,* 20th ed. (Merck & Company, Inc., 2018).

39 *Diagnostic Statistical Manual of Mental Disorders,* 5th ed. (Washington, DC: American Psychiatric Association, 2022.)

FIVE

The Languages of Healing

> Bestowing attention and tender care, by trying every means of
> amendment, in imitation of the best physicians, for neither do
> they cure in one manner only, but when they see the wound
> not yield to the first remedy, they add another, and after that
> again another; and now they use the knife, and now bind up.
> And do thou accordingly, having become a physician of souls.
>
> —John Chrysostom, "Homily XXIX"

The scholar spoke repeatedly of "our common spiritual journey." At an earlier conference I attended on "Healing with Dignity: Spiritual and Pastoral Care in Native America," one attendee of Native American heritage told of being taken away from his mother at age six. He was placed in a boarding school in Canada where priests, nuns, and staff attempted to "whitenize" him. His name was taken away as was his language. His clothes were replaced with proper clothes for white children. His cultural practices were belittled and forbidden. At his boarding school, some children were abused; all the little boys cried themselves to sleep at night.

When I heard the term "our common spiritual journey" for the fifth time in the lecture, I raised my hand during questions and answers. I had to articulate the dissonance of that term, "common," after hearing the narrative of the Native American. The term "spiritual journey" I understood. That it was a "common" spiritual journey, I could not. I was not forcibly removed from my parents as a child. I was not stripped naked of my culture, clothes, identity, and language. I could not identify with this Native American's narrative. I heard the words which were in English, my mother tongue, but I could not process them. Perhaps the horror of what he was sharing cushioned my mind from absorbing them. In that moment, I realized: we do *not* have a common spiritual journey. We may share in common the choice to have a spiritual journey, but there may be no commonalities.

As there are different experiential languages of spiritual journey, there are languages of healing. There are languages of suffering. The healing of an individual is a singular and distinctive phenomenon. The suffering of an individual is unique to them. As those of us in religion and medicine move toward comprehensive care and healing, we would do well to recognize and acknowledge these differing empirical or experient languages. The sufferings described in this book can never be compressed into a single word: suffering. Multivalent healings can never be confined or defined by a noun in the singular: healing. A noun in the singular form refers to one person.

As an example, there is often the singular word: suffering, used in this abstract and general way: the desire to relieve suffering.[1] It is more sensitive and realistic to say: "the desire to relieve sufferings." One word in the singular could never hold the complexity of the continuum of degrees of sufferings or the complexity of pain, agony, misery. Buddhism, for example, describes four sufferings which are universal: birth, aging, sickness, and death. In James Cleary's account of patient Vlad, the fact that a patient's culture can directly impact the degree to which a person suffers is clear. The patient Vlad had incurable brain cancer in Ukraine[2], without the benefit of morphine and other opioids (narcotics).[3] Vlad tried to throw himself out of the hospital window rather that live with excruciating pain and unbearable suffering for which there was no medicinal relief. Vlad's suffering was unbearable. There are levels of sufferings which impact the languages of suffering.

In an earlier version of the *Diagnostic and Statistical Manual* (DSM), there were three types of stressors: acute, episodic acute, and chronic.[4] Although this chart has been eliminated from two subsequent versions of the DSM, it is an example of what would be descriptive and helpful in accessing sufferings.[5]

Ben, a talented young adult, died of an undiagnosed heart condition in 2017 in the family home while his parents were away. In 2023, LeNoir, my friend, and Ben's mother put these words on Facebook on the sixth anniversary of Ben's death:

> How can it be 6 years? Six years empty of his chuckle.
> Six years without hearing, 'Hey, Moms.' Six years without his movie, sports, food and life commentary.
> Six years of memories he is not a part of.
> Certainly, he is IN my memory . . . constantly . . . but these new ones, he's not really a part of . . . only present as the echo of an absence . . . six years. How does time continue without you?
> I still hold you as that sweet baby born on a cold February afternoon and I hold you as that young man you were becoming . . . but

I must also learn to release you . . . into your
now . . . into the embrace of God . . . into the
embrace of eternity . . . into the lively promise
that holds us all. Happy Birthday, Ben.

This suffering of losing a child is catastrophic. To
use the same word for another pain, for example, I am
suffering from a paper cut, is to merge or blur two ends
of a spectrum of suffering. Lenoir and her husband,
Barry, are ministers who preach from the Bible: "This
ancient literature [the Bible] prepares us for 'relentless,
and inexorable and all-encompassing' pain."[6] For Ben's
family, there is no morphine of relief. No pharmaceuticals can heal this wound. Perhaps it will scab, then
form a scar on the soul, but it will not ever go away.
Theirs is a spiritual journey that is unique to them.
Their language of suffering is a dialect of excruciating
pain, on the level of catastrophe. Their faith, hope,
and memories hold them as they rely on the medicines
given by God.[7]

MEDICINE, MIRACLE, AND HEALING

I stood many times before the mural at Houston Methodist Hospital (see color insert). What compels me about
this mural is the stance of Christ the Healer in the middle. Counselors, psychotherapists, and psychiatrists are
taught that the message of arms folded across a person's
chest signifies that they are closed to what is being presented. Christ does not have arms crossed and folded
over his chest which would indicate his rebuff or refusal
to "amendments" to his left and right. Instead, Christ
as Healer is extending his arms to embrace the persons
and procedures represented. There is no opposition by

Christ to the healing through medicine, surgery, and pharmaceutics; in other words, there is no resistance for all healers using every means to find a cure.

The various segments of the mural show a progression in understanding the medical complexity of the healing profession and various significant players in the curing arts. It is a spectrum of "trying every means of amendment" using excerpts from the history of medicine. Many advancements have been made since the mural was created by the Italian artist Bruce Hayes from Florence in 1963.

The left panel begins with Hippocrates and Galen (as the observer faces the mural).

Hippocrates (born 420 BCE) taught that disease was caused naturally, not by superstition and the gods. In other words, disease of the body was not caused by the irritation of the gods such as Asclepius, Greco-Roman God of medicine, and son of Apollo, the god of healing. In a way, the separation of religion (as a pantheon of powerful and controlling gods and goddesses) and medicine may have begun here.

Galen of Pergamon was a Greek physician, surgeon, and philosopher in the Roman Empire, second century CE. He sought to combine philosophical thought with medical practice. Galen believed there was no distinction between the mental and the physical. Thus, we have a beginning of the mind-body connection.

The anatomical drawing of a man is surrounded by animalcules or microorganisms. These microorganisms were first observed by Anthony van Leeuwenhoek, scientist from the Netherlands (1632–1723 CE). His work gave birth to microbiology, and the microscope on the mural represents his contribution. The anatomical drawing illustrates blood circulation; the scalpel nearby honors William Harvey (1578–1657) a doctor from

England who first discovered how blood circulates. On the lower part of Florence Nightingale's skirt, there is the torso of Andreas Vesalius, Flemish physician and anatomist. Vesalius wrote seven books that became *De Humani Corporis Fabrica Libri Septem*, the most comprehensive and influential books on anatomy at that time. Vesalius learned about the body through dissection, a method that for centuries had been considered taboo. He was designated as the father of anatomy.

Florence Nightingale was a social reformer in healthcare nursing, a statistician, and the founder of modern nursing. She was Unitarian, British, and lived in the nineteenth century. Her particular calling was to reduce human suffering. She, like Hippocrates, felt that health was influenced by diet and the environment. She prevented the death of many patients, often soldiers, by her emphasis on hygienic conditions. There was the early awareness that the breakdown of the bodily process occurred with the lack of harmony among the individual, the society, and the environment. The stethoscope represents Rene Theophile Hyacinthe Laennec who in 1816 invented this significant instrument in a hospital in Paris. Now a doctor or nurse could hear the beating of the heart, the rhythm of the veins.

Then, in the center of the mural, is Christ as Healer with arms extended. There is in this portrayal a demeanor of hospitality, security, and openness to faithful connections and medical advances. This receptiveness to various means of healings will be necessary as successful interventions and responses to situational, environmental, and developmental crises present themselves at the hospital. The mural visually brings together spirituality and medical healing and indicates a partnership between the two. The rift between religion and medicine continues to narrow.

The segment of the mural to the right of Christ depicts advances in modern medicine. As the observer faces the mural, to the left of the surgeons is a symbol of a medical theatre. To the right of the surgeons is the portrayal of a body being X-rayed. X-ray was discovered by a German physicist, Wilhelm Conrad Roentgen in 1895, and became "the predecessor of the modern techniques of radiology for both diagnostics and therapy."[8] The row of books represents the "accumulation of knowledge that has brought about the modern 'miracles' of medicine. Apothecary containers symbolize the role of pharmaceutical research" including wonder drugs.[9]

To the extreme right of the mural "are depictions of a heart-lung machine, electronic recorders and monitors and lab components."[10] On the right border is a page from the Bible with Matthew 7:7 featured: "Ask, and it shall be given unto you; seek, and ye shall find; knock, and it shall be opened unto you."[11]

CHRIST AS HEALER, CHRIST OF THE MIRACLES

The Christ of the New Testament engaged in many healings that were seen and described as miracles. In the Gospel of Matthew alone, there are seven healing narratives or miracles: Simon Peter's mother-in-law with a high fever or hyperpyrexia; a man who has leprosy; a man who is paralytic; a man with a withered hand; a woman who is hemorrhaging blood; the dead daughter of a synagogue leader; a centurion's servant who has paralysis; two Gadarene Demoniacs; a man with blindness; two men with blindness on the roadside of Jericho. All of these physical illnesses are cured and witnessed by disciples and townspeople.

Today most Protestant, Orthodox, and Catholic services have prayers for healing. This usually falls under the category "Joys and Concerns." Notably, there are more concerns than joys. In some cases, there are only concerns, and these are mainly prayers for physical healing. Occasionally I see a prayer for the relief of depression or for the removal of fear before surgery. In the event these prayers are visibly or measurably answered, it would be difficult to ferret out the causes of the cure which could be a combination of surgical skill, pharmaceuticals, nursing care, therapeutic intervention, prayer and/or miracle. All of these causes of the cure would be covered by the term introduced earlier as *multivalent healing*.

Many Christians honor the miracles of Christ as Healer in the New Testament. Some claim that Christ still performs them. In her honest struggle with this question, Reverend Debbie Thomas remarks: "I don't struggle with their plausibility. I do struggle with their consequences."[12] Believing in miracles could wound the brokenhearted.[13] What happens when a loved one does not heal or survive an accident? What happens to the hope, the belief system, of those who appear to be denied a miracle? Can their anger, rage, and disappointment in Christ ever be resolved? Thomas struggles with various angles to the question of miracles, but in the end of her powerful essay she confesses: "Yes, I believe in miracles."[14]

In my class discussions, two international students told of firsthand accounts of miraculous healing in their countries of origin: Sierra Leone and Ghana. As grown adults in the modern, Western world, it is not uncommon for us to read stories of miraculous healings and find ourselves hesitant to believe them. But that hesitancy disappears when the student sitting before you has not only seen a miraculous healing, but he himself was the miraculously healed.

Narrative from the interview with Sylvanus Chapman from Sierra Leone:

> I met Sylvanus when he took my Pastoral Theology course at the Perkins School of Theology. His words were delivered with the tune and tenor of his African homeland, every word pronounced with clarity, conviction, and candor. That is exactly how he narrated his story of miraculous healing.
>
> Sylvanus described himself as an accident-prone boy. He played almost every sport and was always active; two ingredients that easily lead to injury. When he was fifteen years old, one particular incident changed everything for Sylvanus. He not only saw the Lord heal through "every means possible," to borrow from Chrysostom, but he chose to give his entire life to the Lord and become an ordained minister, serving the Lord for as long as he lives. This catalyzing incident began when a huge sand truck drove over his left foot. He spent months in the hospital before doctors decided they would need to amputate his foot, believing the foot was becoming "rotten." Sylvanus responded to this news with prayer. Every evening he would fall to his knees in tears, pray to God, and promise God that if he could use his two feet again, he would use them for God. This was the promise he made again and again. One night, Sylvanus had a dream that his

deceased mother was holding his hand and walking with him through their village— Sylvanus walking on both of his feet. In this dream, Sylvan was surrounded by leaves that he knew were used for healings. After Sylvanus told his father about this dream, Sylvanus's father wasted no time taking him back to their home village. He spent only one week back home in their village before everything changed. The men in his village would hold him as the boiled leaves were placed on his feet. He says this treatment was hell; however, within just a week he was once again playing soccer in his village. He had been healed. While Sylvanus does acknowledge the use of the boiled leaves, he ultimately credits prayer and the Miraculous Healer with his divine healing.

Narrative from the interview with Richard Pokoo from Ghana:

Before sharing his story with me, Richard posed a question that seemed serendipitously fitting. "Can we pray?" Richard asked. The moment felt sacred and indescribably apt. Before telling the story of the miracle he witnessed, Richard wanted to thank the Miracle Maker, the God of every story, including his own. Richard's story began in Ghana, where he was raised in the Ghana Methodist Church before immigrating to the United States in 1999. He was an active member of his youth group in Ghana and their evangelistic ministry throughout the Western Region.

The mission of their evangelism group was to trek into the remote villages that had not yet been reached by missionaries and the Word of God. It was precisely in the midst of this evangelistic outreach that Richard saw God reach in and do the miraculous.[15]

Before departing for these outreach missions, Richard and his youth group would spend time—at least one whole week in prayer and fasting—confessing their need for strength and the power of the Holy Spirit. For Richard's youth group, this habitual practice was not the result of mere conviction or Scriptural inspiration but it was brought about by the recognition of the demonic forces in the African villages; forces they knew they might encounter. They wanted to be as prepared as possible and being well prepared meant having spent countless hours looking up to God for strength instead of looking within. Once prepared, Richard's group would then journey to a remote village and spend at least three nights with the people of the village.

On the particular mission where Richard saw God perform the miraculous, the journey initially began like any other. When they got to the village, they went into a classroom and prayed, committing the community "into the hands of God." They prepared to show the village that they were there as community partners, those who were following the biblical mandate to love one's neighbor as oneself, in the hope that toward the end of their outreach they would have a good turnout at the crusade. (In this context, an African crusade is similar to what Americans would think of as a Billy Graham style revival.) And yet, during this time of preparation Richard's group realized this wasn't an ordinary mission. During their time of prayer, God revealed to one of Richard's sisters-in-Christ that three people were going to die in the village—that very night. They went on with their preparations, completely forgetting about the prophesy . . . until it began to come true. When they heard a man sobbing and banging on the door, they learned that a woman who had recently given birth was no longer responding. Everyone said she was dead. The man had approached Richard's group because he knew they could pray for her to come back to life. Richard then took a few people with him to the house where the woman was. Richard saw both mother and baby, and his heart was filled with compassion. "This mother cannot leave this baby," Richard thought. Richard and his group began to call upon God for the miraculous, praying "for about three hours without even knowing we were praying," Richard recounted. Suddenly, there was a prophetic revelation telling them to grab a container of water and pray over it. They were instructed to then pour it over the woman. As the water fell upon the woman, she came back to life. Richard then washed her face, and she regained all of her strength. Richard and his group looked at one another and wondered,

"Is this real? What are we seeing?" They were seeing the miraculous.

In the mural at Houston Methodist Hospital, the center figure, Christ the Healer, represents the One who performed miracles. The true encounters described by Sylvanus and Richard are examples of contemporary examples of this. At the same time, the relevance of the extending arms of Christ the Healer is an embrace of other means and modes of cure.

Some struggle with the consequences of miracles, not for those who receive a miracle but for those who do not. Rev. Dr. Wil Gafney's sermon on "Gonna Take a Miracle" develops this theme of "unanswered prayer" for a miracle. "In our world, talk of miracles can be dangerous; they are food for starving people. The folk talking the most about miracles are often frauds, seeking to defraud those most desperately in need of a healing or saving touch. Real miracles are unpredictable. They are not dependent on us. And yet, Jesus tells the woman with the vaginal hemorrhage that her faith has saved her."[16] With sensitivity and awareness of those who desperately need a miracle and do not receive it, Gafney still affirms her belief in miracles. This is not an uncommon struggle. It is the challenge of trusting the truth of the miraculous while struggling with the fact that not all will receive this intervention and gift.

God works with the world, and our prayers for healing can be in partnership with God.[17] Marjorie Hewitt Suchocki writes: "These prayers can make the difference between reversing a not-yet-irreversible illness or not; therefore, God bids us to pray."[18] At some point, whether through accident, illness, disease, or age, we will all die. God cannot or does not prevent this. Suchocki uses the example of her son-in-law, Butch, who died at thirty-eight of leukemia despite fervent prayers on his behalf. Prayers for his healing were not answered but "are now being answered through the health of his young family."[19] She sees one form of healing as the ability of his survivors—in due time—to embrace life lovingly again.[20] When asked if miracles still occur, she answers: I believe.

I recently asked a Lutheran pastor if he believed prayers were efficacious in healing. His father, also a Lutheran pastor, had been killed as a result of an automobile accident while his son was a young boy. This son, now retired, told how his uncle, a prominent surgeon, had been able to have his father airlifted from the site of the accident to a hospital in the family's hometown of Lincoln, Nebraska. The father lived for six days while his family and his church members gathered and prayers for his recovery were said. He died. I asked again if this pastor thought prayers made any difference. He answered, "Yes. We were given six more days with him."

Someone who has been in and out of many hospitals offered this important critique. She read the early draft of this book. "A lot of the stories you present in the book are of bodily healings. Many of us, however, cannot relate to those stories. That does not mean that those stories are not significant or needed, but it means that they aren't comprehendible by those of us who live with congenital or chronic conditions that remain unhealed. I spent years of my childhood praying to be healed, and then I stopped praying for that. I didn't give up on the idea that God could heal, but I began to realize that for me, spiritual healing was greater than physical healing. Sure, God could show his power to do the miraculous by healing me physically (the bargaining chip I used in many prayers), but perhaps the miraculous is also shown in the resilience and perseverance to get up every day in pain and steward this body that is a gift. I think the spiritual healing that enables one to lovingly accept and steward their diseased or disabled embodiment is also miraculous. And in this sense, chaplains, ministers, physicians of faith, all of whom are physicians of the soul, are just as important if not more important than mere physicians of the body. They enter in when medicine and medical practices have essentially reached their limits. I think acknowledging this reality might be a way to do two things. First, you could reach an audience that can't grasp miraculous, physical healings. Second, you could tie the message of the book together by articulating the significant, crucial role of a physician of the soul when physicians of the body have lost their power in terminal or progressive cases." I agree and am grateful for this incisive critique.

Miracles. For those of us who affirm modern day miracles, we still have the problem of partially answered or unanswered prayer when a healing does not happen. I have experienced that. I prayed for our son from the day he came to us through adoption. He was born in my heart, and I loved him more than my own life. He was exposed in utero to crack cocaine which resulted in specific challenges as he grew into manhood. At twenty-six, he pulled his life together and had a wonderful job, a family, and a child on the way.

The call came on a Saturday morning; he had been killed in a single car accident. Having pulled a double work shift, he had fallen asleep and hit a utility pole. Shock and numbness took over. Then came rage—at God. My husband and I have each served the church and God for over thirty years. Couldn't God have given our son a few inches between his car and the utility pole? Just a few inches. Couldn't he have veered into a bush or wooden fence nearby? Couldn't God have done this for us? I know the woundedness of receiving no miracle.

Nevertheless, I stand by the narratives of Richard and Sylvanus. I am exceedingly grateful in villages that lacked medical doctors, clinics, and hospitals, God used another way to heal. I will always have a scab on my heart for my unanswered prayer, yet I still believe. This is my unique (not common) spiritual journey. I believe God can act in the world in healings (spiritual and bodily) and through miracles. The miracle could be the resilience and perseverance to keep going when there is no cure or healing. Ultimately, as in the case of our son, I believe "there is a health that is deeper than death."[21]

INNOVATIONS IN MEDICINE AND MINISTRY

Innovations and advances in the link between medicine and religion are ongoing if not burgeoning. The annual meeting of The American Academy of Religion now features a unit on "Religions, Medicines, and Healing." The bifurcation of religion and medicine is lessening as the awareness of the connectivity between body-mind-soul is increasing. The American Academy of Religion also added a unit in 2023 titled "Innovations in Chaplaincy & Spiritual Care" which focuses on chaplains and spiritual care in healthcare settings. Hospitals are realizing the healing advantage of spiritual care to the mending of the mind, the solace of the soul, and the benefit to the body.

If Bruce Hayes, the artist of the mural titled "Extending Arms of Christ," was able to extend the mural, he would need to add advances in the healing arts. Since the creation of this tableau at Houston Methodist Hospital in 1963, there have been numerous breakthroughs and developments. A few of these are as follows: psychedelic-assisted therapy; partnerships between chaplains and medical professionals; spiritual quests for a meaning to continue living; Adverse Religious Experiences (ARE); healing soul wounds; compassion in healthcare.

Psychedelic-assisted therapy

One of the most prominent examples of innovations in healing is psychedelic-assisted therapy. For example, researchers at the Emory Center for Psychedelics and Spirituality for Mind, Body, Soul in Atlanta are exploring the use of psychedelic-assisted therapy as are established universities such as Yale University, hospitals such as Johns Hopkins, and cancer centers such as Aquilino Cancer Center in Rockville, MD. Using the psychedelic Psilocybin, a chemical found in certain mushrooms, tests have shown a lessening if not elimination of different psychiatric disorders such as OCD, anxiety, eating disorders, addiction, depression, anorexia nervosa, and end-of-life fear. After taking one pill of Psilocybin, those in treatment described revelatory, mystical, or transcendental experiences that always result in positive well-being, a loss of fear, a sense that the universe is in good hands, and healing of painful memories. A pill containing Psilocybin is taken only once or twice in a lifetime.[22]

Partnerships between chaplains and medical professionals

Chaplaincy and spiritual caregivers are expanding their ministries into healthcare and medical settings. Medical professionals are extending hospitality to this expansion. Wendy Cadge's *Spiritual Care: The Everyday Work of Chaplains*[23] is built on her interviews and ethnographic research with sixty-six chaplains in the

Boston area, following them down hospital hallways and cavernous corridors. As chaplains and spiritual caregivers "work around death"[24] and "broker end-of-life issues serving as midwives to death"[25], the reality of the holding space, the liminal moments, and the in-between-places where chaplains and spiritual caregivers work are clearly discerned. As chaplains are included more in palliative care, their contribution to the relief of pain will be recognized.

Spiritual quests for a meaning to continue living

This next example is not a recent innovation, but unique forms of it can bridge spirituality and medicine. This technique may be offered by ministers, chaplains, imams, priests, rabbis, and shamans. It is the process of finding and articulating the meaning of one's life in the midst of sufferings. It was developed by Dr. Viktor Frankl, a medical doctor in Vienna, Austria, while imprisoned. This positive technique was used by Viktor Frankl while a prisoner in the Tuerkheim Concentration Camp in 1944 during World War II. Having lost his parents, his wife Tilly and their unborn son, and his brother in Auschwitz-Birkenau, Theresienstadt, and Bergen-Belsen camps, Frankl was in misery. He contracted typhoid fever, and knew he would die without medication and with continual work in the bitter, cold winds of the work sites. He wrote: "I forced my thoughts to turn to another subject. Suddenly, I saw myself standing on the platform of a well-lit and pleasant lecture room. In front of me sat an attentive audience on comfortable upholstered seats. I was giving a lecture on the psychology of the concentration camp! All that oppressed me at that moment became objective, seen and described from a remote viewpoint of science. By this method I succeeded somehow in rising about the situation, above the sufferings of the moment, and I observed them as if they were already of the past."[26]

Frankl lived until 1997, spoke to many attentive audiences, and developed a therapeutic approach termed logotherapy. Whereas psychoanalysis focused on the pleasure principle and on the status drive or will-to-power, Frankl emphasized the will-to-meaning in *logotherapy*. What does life expect from us? What gives us meaning even throughout horrific suffering? These are questions for the physicians of the soul and for their patients and parishioners. John Chrysostom used rhetoric in the form of therapeutic *logos*, "directed towards teaching the individual how to regulate their soul in regard to desire and affect/*pathos*, in large part through attainment of the correct mindset."[27] This was a rational therapy likened to medicine. Pain and imminent death can induce a search for meanings.

Adverse Religious Experience (ARE)

For many years, literature and treatments have been developing around Adverse Childhood Experiences (ACE) such as abuse, malnourishment, poverty, neglect, violence, homelessness, torture, and other harmful treatment or life experience.[28] Childhood is considered to be from zero to seventeen years. Now researchers are becoming increasingly aware of Adverse Religious Experiences which can impact any age. Daren Slade writes: "AREs are any experience of a religious belief, practice, or structure that undermines an individual's sense of safety or autonomy/and or negatively impacts their physical, social, emotional, relational, or psychological wellbeing."[29] Religious Trauma (RT) refers to lasting adverse effects after an ARE.

Examples of Religious Trauma can be related to a misuse of the Bible: "He who spares the rod hates his son, but he who loves him is diligent to discipline him." (Proverbs 13:24) This verse has been taken to literal extremes and resulted in injury, even death. Another passage of Scripture that causes trauma is the interpretation of the ancient household codes in Ephesians 5: 22-33, where the wife is to be submissive to the husband. This text has been distorted to support battering of women. The key verse to the whole pericope or biblical passage is always overlooked in these cases: "Submit to one another out of reverence for Christ." (Eph 5:21)

Healing Soul Wounds

To heal soul wounds is to deal with historical trauma. Native American therapist Eduardo Duran states boldly: "I have not been able to find any acknowledgement of historical trauma in the DSM-V and therefore feel safe in making the assumption that diagnosing Native People is not an accurate process."[30] The uniqueness of healing the soul wounds of Native Americans, according to Duran, is to move fourteen generations into the healing process, seven generations back and seven generations forward. Everything we do affects every generation. Therefore, if one does not find healing in his or her generation, the soul wounding will be passed down to their children, grandchildren, great-grandchildren, and four more generations. Healing begins with the acknowledgement of the power of God. Just as Christ befriended the demoniac, so must disease and wounding be befriended, shape-shifted or transformed, and turned by the Spirit into a life force. "Godding" happens as sacramental psychotherapy takes place between therapist and client. Dreams are significant in the process, the memory of good things in one's DNA need to be acknowledged, the support of the community is invaluable, and forgiveness comes into play. A Lakota

Native American term is that of the "hollow bone." The practitioner sucks out the disease or soul wound so that the one suffering may become like a hollow bone with the spirit of life flowing through. Compassion keeps the disease or soul wound from sticking to you. Duran writes: "It is important to note that the soul-wounding process has left an emptiness in the soul of the wounded person. That emptiness of soul or spirit is seeking to fill the void with spirit."[31] He also reminds us that when we wound Mother Earth, we hurt ourselves as well.

Compassion in healthcare

According to an analysis offered by Professor Joshua Hordern, there is a shift coming in healthcare that could be described as more person-centered than patient-centered. There will be a type of de-medicalization in the relationship between medical personnel and patient. Hordern says:

> There is a relational vision of human persons, which, like yeast, is leavening the biomedical discourse in such a way as to make a full-bodied healthcare rise out from under the anemic, de-localised "medical gaze", with the benefits of evidence-based medicine but also with a newly enriched appreciation of the significance for healthcare of people's narratives, values, and places.[32]

New research out of The Catholic University of America is highlighting the need and the barriers to providing hospice and palliative care for homeless and vulnerably housed individuals (HVHI). Barriers include lack of electricity and running water, food, safety, and social support. Compassion in healthcare is extending to the most vulnerable of patients through research and legislation.[33]

Compassion in healthcare is extending to rural communities like Clay County, West Virginia. As one of only two doctors in the county, Dr. Kimberly Becher is a family practitioner who visits "children in their living rooms to vaccinate them, organizes food drives and administers Suboxone to treat opioid addiction."[34] Becher works for Community Care of West Virginia, a federally qualified health center.[35] West Virginia is at the top of most lists for poverty, obesity poor health outcomes, coronary disease, depression, shortest life expectancy. Most residents live in a food desert with no public transportation in the county and no hospital. On April 17, 2021, Becher felt she was having a heart attack, got to an emergency room, and was diagnosed with takotsubo cardiomyopathy (sometimes called broken heart syndrome). Her life as a rural physician had to slow down. In her new role, she is developing "a support group for rural physicians through the Robert C. Byrd Center for Rural Health at Marshall University."[36]

In the predicted shift in healthcare toward more compassion in the treatment of patients, we are coming back to the advice of Chrysostom: "Bestowing attention and tender care by trying every means of amendment, in imitation of the best physicians" . . . like Dr. Kimberly Becher.

MEDICINE AS MINISTRY, MINISTRY AS MEDICINE

I began this book as something of a response to Dr. Margaret Mohrmann's work on *Medicine as Ministry*. Here is an example of an anxious United Methodist minister in Memphis, Tennessee, facing orthopedic surgery when her long-time cardiologist offers ministry to her:

I was having my hip replacement in Methodist Hospital Germantown. The surgical receptionist called me to say the person scheduled
before me had not shown up. I hurried to the
hospital. The staff worked fast to prepare me.
In the midst of the preparations, in walked
my cardiologist into the holding room. All
eyes were on him. Two nurses began asking
me questions while starting my I-V. Before
I could answer, the distinguished doctor
announced: "I need to pray with her. She is
one of my patients." He grabbed my hand.
He prayed for the doctors, nurses, my peace,
and God's care over me. Then, he was gone.
He came by my room twice while I was in
the hospital. The two surgical nurses said:
"Is that the doctor . . . .? He is pretty stern,
but he is nice with you." They could tell how
much he cared. He has done that one other
time. After office visits, he prays for me.

He as a physician offered healing prayer, pastoral presence, and ministry to someone going through the anxiety of facing surgery. The fact that the patient prepping
for surgery in this case is a seasoned minister makes the
exchange even more poignant. Medicine as ministry.

The following and closing example is that of a
minister offering "the medicine of God" to a fatherless
child. This positive transformation of the boy's negative
identity is what those of us who are therapists attempt.
This story was told to me by Dr. Fred Craddock in his
retirement. I recorded it, and Dr. Craddock was very
pleased. He said he had heard people give faulty ren-
ditions of his story, and he would be happy to set the
record straight.[37]

My wife and I were on vacation in Gatlinburg and over to our table came this old man who was a greeter and, I learned later, a part owner of The Black Bear Inn. He said "Good evening," and we said, "Good evening," and he asked where we were from; we were at that time in Oklahoma. And then he asked what I did. I was getting a little irritated because he was a stranger, and he didn't need all that. But when I told him I was a minister, he said, "I have a story about a minister" and pulled out a chair and sat down at our table. Uninvited by the way, but it's his business. I thought he was going to tell a joke; everybody has a joke about a minister. I thought, he's going to tell one, and I would pretend I had never heard it and smile, and he would go away.

At any rate, he said, "I was born not far from here, out from the village of Cosby, in a place called Laurel Springs. My mother was not married. The children at school made fun of me. I ate my lunch alone. I hid during recess because they said ugly things to me. When I went to town, people looked at my mother and me. I just figured they were trying to make guesses as to who was my father. So I had a very painful childhood. In the course of it, I started going—about middle school age—to Laurel Springs Christian Church back in the woods; it had kerosene lamps. There was an old preacher there with a long beard, a chiseled face, and a deep voice. I liked to hear him preach but I didn't want to be embarrassed. I would just go for the sermon and rush out. I did that for some time. One day some of the people gathered in the aisle, and I couldn't get by, and I felt this hand on my shoulder, and I looked around and I could see the face and the beard of the preacher. I was scared to death because I was always afraid of being embarrassed in public. He stared at me as though he was trying to guess what man in the community was my father. After he looked at me carefully, he said, 'Boy you are a child of . . .' He paused there. I just froze. 'Boy, you are a child of . . . God. I see a striking resemblance.' He patted me on the shoulders and said, 'Go claim your inheritance.' That was really the first day of my life."

I said to the greeter, "your name again?" He said, "[a governor, twice-elected]." I remembered my father talking about the people of Tennessee twice electing [this man] as governor of the state although he was called publicly, especially by the political opposition, the "bastard governor." My father said, "The people of Tennessee twice elected a bastard governor."

The former governor wanted his story told. He said to me, "My papers are at the University of Tennessee and will be published after my death, and I have asked that my story be told as the preface of encouragement to other children born here in the mountains, children of 'questionable background.'"

That was [the former governor]. It was that expression, "you are a child of God, I see a striking resemblance. Go claim your inheritance," that stays with me. That was one of the most moving experiences I ever had. It came as such a surprise especially when I was resisting his even being there, interrupting our evening meal. That was quite a moment. It is a true and remarkable story.

In this encounter, a minister offers a repositioning or renaming. The title "child of God" overcame the demeaning label, "bastard child." The nomenclature "child of God" is the essential, definite, pervasive, and ultimate demarcation of The-One-to-Whom Christians belong. It can supplant biological ties and relationships. The label "child of God" can be transformative and eventually healing, as it was in the case of the twice-elected governor of Tennessee who began to "claim his inheritance" as well as his identity. Reimaging one's self as child of God can not only impact present functioning, but can reconfigure the way the past is viewed and fortify a person for the future.

Here is a minister offering healing through image repositioning which transformed this young boy's self-identity. This is the goal of much professional therapy particularly when trauma is involved. Ministry as medicine.

NOTES

1   Robert Fine and Jack Levison, eds., *The Pursuit of Life: The Promise and Challenge of Palliative Care* (University Park, PA: The Pennsylvania State University Press, 2023).

2   James Cleary, "The Robin Hood of Opioids: Palliative Care in the Underdeveloped World" in *The Pursuit of Life: The Promise and Challenge of Palliative Care*, eds. Robert Fine and Jack Levison (University Park, PA: The Pennsylvania State University Press, 2023), 157.

3   80 per cent of the world's population lacks access to morphine.

4   *Diagnostic and Statistical Manual*, 3rd ed. Revised, (Washington, DC: The American Psychiatric Association, 1987), 11.

5   *Diagnostic and Statistical Manual*, 5th ed. Revised.

6   *Diagnostic and Statistical Manual*, 5th ed. Revised.

7   Matt II:16 which is the basis for Chrysostom's"Homily IX," page 158. There are a number of mentions of the medicines given by God such as moderation, salvation, almsgiving, the hearing of the Scriptures, etc. In this case, I believe the medicine to these parents pertains to the birth, death, and subsequent resurrection of Christ: "And what is marvelous, thou wilt see death destroyed by death." Homily II, Matthew 1.1.

8   Buddy Scott, "Arms of Christ Mural Embraces Medical Profession History" in THE FACTS: Covering Brazoria County—Where Texas Began (Clute, Texas, 12/31/2011). Scott is a religion columnist whose father introduced him to the mural when he was a teenager. I am indebted to Scott for identifying several items on the mural.

9   Scott, "Arms of Christ Mural."

10   Scott, "Arms of Christ Mural.".

11   The opposite side features a scroll on the edge.

12   Debbie Thomas, "Why and How I Believe in Miracles" in *The Christian Century*, June (2023): 33–34.

13   Thomas, "Why and How I Believe in Miracles," 34.

14   Thomas, "Why and How I Believe in Miracles," 33.

15   Paul Glen Grant, *Healing and Power in Ghana: Early Indigenous Expressions of Christianity* (Waco: Baylor University Press, 2020), 181, footnote 80. Grant traces faith healings from ailments to German Pietism and Pentecostalism in the first decade of the twenty-first century. The resurrection of Kwame Akwatia, a young boy who died December 28, 1858, parallels the account told by Richard. See pages 228–32.

16   The Reverend Dr. Wil Gafney, "Gonna Take A Miracle," sermon preached on February 5, 2023. All Saints Episcopal Church Kaua'I, Year A, *A Women's Lectionary for the Whole Church*, see wilgafney.com.

17 Suchocki, Marjorie Hewitt Suchocki, *In God's Presence: Theological Reflections on Prayer* (St. Louis: Chalice Press, 1996), 57.

18 Suchocki, *In God's Presence*, 59.

19 Suchocki, *In God's Presence*, 63.

20 Suchocki, *In God's Presence*, 63.

21 Suchocki, *In God's Presence*, 60.

22 "How to Change Your Mind," narrated by Michal Pollan, author of the book by the same name. This information comes from the miniseries on Netflix, episode 2, and conversations with colleagues.

23 Wendy Cadge, *Spiritual Care: The Everyday Work of Chaplains* (Oxford University Press, 2022)

24 Cadge, *Spiritual Care*, 16.

25 Cadge, *Spiritual Care.* 125.

26 Viktor E. Frankl, preface to *The Doctor and the Soul: From Psychotherapy to Logotherapy*, 3rd ed. (New York: Penguin Random House, 1955), xiii.

27 Wendy Mayer, "Shaping the Sick Soul: Reshaping the Identity of John Chrysostom," in *Christians Shaping Identity from the Roman Empire to Byzantium: Studies inspired by Pauline Allen*, Supplements to Vigilae Christianae 132 (Leiden: Brill, 2015), 159.

28 Roberts, Matthias, "How to Find Healing from Religious Trauma," Sojourners magazine, September-October issue, 2023.

29 Darren M. Slade, "Adverse Religious Experiences (AREs) vs. Religious Trauma (RT): An Important Distinction," (Global Center for Religious Research Academic Institute, Denver, CO, August 8, 2022). www.-gcrr-org.cdn.amproject.org.

30 Eduardo Duran, *Healing the Soul Wound: Trauma-Informed Counseling for Indigenous Communities*, 2nd ed. (New York and London: Teachers College Press, 2019), 33. The DSM-V is the *Diagnostic and Statistical Manual* in a fifth edition.

31 Duran, *Healing the Soul Wound*, 78

32 Joshua Hordern, *Compassion in Healthcare: Pilgrimage, Practice, and Civic Life* (Oxford: Oxford University Press, 2020), 2–3.

33 Hannah Loring Murphy Buc, "Ain't Never Been Cared For: A Grounded Theory of Receiving Hospice and Palliative Care for Homeless and Vulnerably Housed Individuals," (PhD Diss., Conway School of Nursing, The Catholic University in America, 2023), 4.

34 Oliver Whang, "A Rural Doctor Gave Her All. Then Her Heart Broke." *New York Times*, September 19, 2022. https://www.nytimes.com/2022/09/19/health/doctor-burnout-west-virginia.html

35 Whang, "A Rural Doctor Gave Her All"

36 Whang, "A Rural Doctor Gave Her All"

37 Fred Craddock, in a recorded interview with Jeanne Stevenson-Moessner and printed in *The Spirit of Adoption: At Home in God's Family* (Louisville: Westminster John Knox Press, 2003), 10–11. Reprinted with permission.

Conclusion

"Physician of the soul" as a term has been the hinge of this book. The term is borrowed from the writings of John Chrysostom (fourth century) and applied to the context of the twenty-first century with application to all faith traditions including Christianity. The nomenclature "physician of the soul" is utilized to make an intentional connection with physicians of the body and physicians of the mind. There is a growing awareness and hospitality to the impact of spirituality on healing. Chaplaincy and spiritual caregivers are expanding their ministries into healthcare and medical settings which include military, fire department, hospice, and community settings.[1] There is an openness in medicine to this influx of religion which is in accord with Chrysostom's emphasis on "using every means of cure." In this book, the term *multivalent healing* has represented this openness to avenues of healing and context of care.

The separation of medicine and religion has been traced to Hippocrates, often referred to as "the father of modern medicine." At that time, religion was dominated by a pantheon of gods and goddesses who, when angry at humankind, would inflict disease, illness, even death on humans. As increasing knowledge was gained by dissecting, treating, and exploring the body in a primitive way, the causes of disease, illness, and death were seen as located in viruses, infections, bacteria, fungi, parasites, external injury to the body, and aging. Medicine and Religion became separated from one another. There were exceptions to this statement. For example, indigenous cultures where the healer was also the priest or religious leader.

In this book, the growing partnership between medicine and religion has been shown. This has been motivated, in part, by the conviction that the body-mind-soul are interconnected in a way that involves sickness and health. The terms physician of the body, physician of the mind, and physician of the soul undergird and exemplify that interrelationship. The Hippocratic Oath supports this connection. "Or in the words of the Hippocratic Oath: the physician must protect [the] patient from the mischief and injustice which [they] may inflict upon [themselves] if [the diet] is not properly chosen. [The physician] must be a physician of the soul no less than the body; [the physician] must not overlook the moral implications of his or [her] actions, nor even the negative indices to be watched; for the regimen followed by a person concerns [their] bodily and psychic constitution."[1]

A result of the pandemic has been a lessening of the division between medicine and religion. Incredible teamwork occurred in hospitals across the nation as medical professionals and religious professionals worked overtime to care for those infected with the virus. All hands were needed, especially at the bedside of the gravely ill or dying. I doubt there were few times when a physician of the body ever doubted the need for physicians of the soul. Covid-19 and the pandemic raised universal questions about the search for meaning and the will to live.

The Corona era challenged many people to face their mortality as friends and family became ill, as death took many in those early weeks of the outbreak. The scenes on television showed stretchers in makeshift tents in parking lots of hospitals with no more room. Just as a Clinical Pastoral Education student or chaplain intern faces mortality while responding to a code blue and watching death take over, so did many people face the possibility of their mortality for the first time. It is no wonder that in the post Corona era, increasing numbers of Americans are taking early retirement, changing jobs, spending more time at home and with family. They had to face the question Viktor Frankl faced: What does life expect from us? What gives us meaning even throughout horrific suffering? The rise in suicides could be related to some of these questions—mixed with the loneliness isolated people faced.

Images are absorbed. Concepts are learned. Concepts can be changed through education.

The only way to change an image is to shatter it.[2]

The images we absorbed during the Covid-19 pandemic were those of masked doctors and nurses desperately caring for beds of patients lodged in hallways. The images of the slow murder of George Floyd gave us indelible depictions of racial brutality. The images of women in court testifying to sexual abuse— whether the Olympic gymnasts or aspiring actresses of Hollywood—will never be erased because we absorb images. This absorption of images gives my field of Practical and Pastoral Theology much work to do as we seek to shatter evil and replace it with justice and well-being.

As pastoral caregivers give attention to the languages of suffering, the languages of evil, and the languages of spiritual journey, we can only fine-tune our listening to the sounds of the soul.

Physicians of the soul work with a sensitivity to narratives of harm that a person may carry. It is our vocation to help create a safe and caring environment. For some, the hospital is a frightening place especially if relatives have died there or if the individual has undergone such procedures as chemotherapy or a rape exam there. I offered a credo of care-givers that contains boundaries, safety measures, and sacred responsibilities for those giving care.

Religion is often conceived or misconceived as having an arsenal of sin and damnation. John Chrysostom emphasized the virtues in life, and in related fashion; I offered a Trinity of Virtues as a way to proceed. Building on the three greatest Biblical virtues, we have a triad of love of God, love of neighbor, and love of self. Thus, the opposite of the last virtue is not pride, but the degradation and shame of one's self, the hatred of one's body, the inability to see oneself as a beloved child of God. There is much work to be done of renaming the "seven deadly sins" which has been traditionally defined by men. This emphasis on sins has cluttered the grace and healing that can be offered through religion.

A recent example may offer an model of comprehensive and restorative care by both institutions of medicine and religion. One of my greatest honors was the access I had as an ordained minister to hospitals that were closed to visitors, including family. The baby of my daughter's best friend became gravely ill and was taken by ambulance from a midwestern town to the University of Iowa Children's Hospital in Iowa City. The young parents were allowed to stay with the baby during the week and a half of medical intervention, but no other family members were allowed in the Covid-closed hospital. The one exception was an ordained minister and that became me. The young couple allowed me to pray over their infant son at the end of each visit. I drove almost daily the three hours round trip to the University hospital with changes of clothes for them, baby's favorite toys, food they craved, raspberries for the sick child (his favorite food), and so it went. It was providential that I was on research leave in the Midwest. The child recovered in time. I take no credit for that, but the parents were never alone in their fear, never cut off from home, never without their favorite sweater or hoodie. My ministry was simply a pastoral presence, and that was honored time and again by the medical staff of a university hospital.

I have driven that same route from the midwestern city to Iowa City since then for other reasons. It has seemed like a long three hours. By contrast, on the days I drove the distance to be with a precious couple hovering over a very sick child, it did not feel long. On the way there, I remember the time as a spiritual preparation and retreat. The gorgeous landscape of fall in Iowa nurtured me. The time with the family was a privilege that humbled me. On the way home, I would sometimes stop to wander in a lavish plant nursery where I was inspired by God's creation of flowers and vegetables in so many colors. Inevitably, a plant went home with me as did a sense of my vocation.

If you were to ask me about the healing of this young child, I would say he had the best of physicians who were attentive and tried every means of cure. The chief pediatric cardiologist often brought a team of child specialists in with him on rounds in the mornings to discuss options and alternative approaches. The nurses were diligent, caring, understanding of the stresses on families of sick children, tender with the IVs and shots, and ultimately loving. They never gave me the sense I was in the way. It seemed we were a team. I never stayed longer than my physician father had trained me to stay.

How would I account for the healing of this child? Surely, if we were to quantify and break up components into fractions, the team of physicians would have a high number. The nurses' number would be high as would the pharmaceutical interventions. It would not be possible for me to quantify or to ferret out the answer. I would need to factor in the chaplain at the university hospital whom I called to meet the ambulance and who followed them to the emergency room. I would need to include all the ways that hospital room was made a holding environment for the young parents. Yes, I did pray along with a vast network of others who asked God for healing. I will never have a quantitative answer, only a qualitative response as I have given.

I do not mind coming to the end with the awareness of how much I still do not know or will never know. For this matter of healing and the contributions of religion and medicine to healing is much more complex and wonderous than a book can reveal. I can minister with a qualitative answer because I know illness has many faces: scarred, afraid, discarded, shattered, hungry, and covered with rashes, to name a few. Our role as physicians of the soul is to care, to accompany, to attend, and in some cases, to cure. I also know that the journey to get to those who need us, regardless of the time and terrain it takes, will never seem too long.

NOTES

1 Edelstein, Ludwig. Ancient Medicine: Selected Papers of Ludwig Edelstein, eds. Owsei Temkin and Lilian Temkin, (Baltimore & London: The Johns Hopkins University Press, 1987), p.25.

2 Nelle Morton, *The Journey Is Home* (Boston: Beacon Press, 1985 reprint), 31. Nelle Morton was a Christian educator and a member of the Fellowship of Southern Churchmen who fought segregation in the South of the USA.

Epilogue

Self-disclosure is hard for me given the way I was trained as a psychotherapist. It is only allowed if it would clearly benefit the listener, the client. As an author and theologian, I am only disclosing something very personal which may give you, the reader, a reason behind my desire to write this book.

In the summer of 2021, my husband, daughter, and I were driving through Iowa to take our young grand-daughters home after their week with us. I realized I was having a full menstrual period many years after menopause. We dropped the girls off and headed to a "fully-equipped" hospital in Carrollton, Iowa. The signage outside said "fully-equipped." That weekend, the hospital had lent out its only ultrasound machine to a rural hospital. I was examined and told to see an OB-GYN upon returning home. I did.

The OB-GYN examined me and requested a cancer antigen (CA125) blood test. My score was slightly elevated, and the OB-GYN suspected cancer. I was sent to an oncologist who ordered several specific tests and scans, sometimes twice. This took almost a week.

The day came for me to get the results. My family was out-of-town so I asked a dear friend, Dr. Bonnie Sue Lewis, to go with me to the cancer clinic to hear the results. I was afraid I might be stunned by the diagnosis and wanted a second set of ears.

We entered the waiting room. I saw many patients wearing bandanas over their heads. I remember thinking: that could be me some day. We sat in a corner of the large room, and Bonnie Sue asked if she could pray. Of course, I said "yes." While she was praying, I had the distinct sensation of something warm like wax or paraffin being poured over my entire body from head to feet. It was not only a warming sensation, it was comforting and soothing. I heard Bonnie Sue say "Amen." Then, my name was called by the receptionist. We went to an examination room.

I sat on the examination table while Bonnie Sue was in a chair nearby. We waited. Suddenly, the Oncologist burst through the door with a sheaf of papers and folders about seven or eight inches thick. She dropped them on her metal desk and looked up at me. "They are clear," she announced with a slight tone of incredulity. She repeated the results, I gave a stunned "thank-you." Then Bonnie Sue and I left.

To this day, I can remember the experience of being cocooned in a warm, molding substance. It is as real to me as the fact that I am sitting in a chair, in my dining room, writing these words on my laptop. This is why I started with the story of Mrs. Mattingly's Miracle (1824) in Chapter One, included a modern-day miracle (Anne O'Connell, 1975), added the two narratives of Richard Pokoo and Sylvanus Chapman, and disclosed mine. The term *multivalent healing*, I believe, includes accounts such as these.

Harder for me to understand is why a good and all-powerful God would allow some to be healed and others not—by using every means of cure. Why would a loving God allow an innocent baby to die? What benevolent God would permit a child to suffer unto death? Why would a compassionate God let guiltless bystanders be shot and die? Why would children be born with congenital limb anomalies? Why would one in four children "live with at least one chronic condition: heart disease, stroke, cancer, diabetes, asthma, cerebral palsy, muscular dystrophy, and so on?"[1] This agonizing question is called theodicy. Theodicy is the issue or argument that tries to resolve the benevolence, omniscience, and omnipotence of God with examples of evil, like the ones I described above. Other examples would involve evil experienced by groups, nations, clans, and tribes.

Some have tried to answer this question of theodicy. In his book, *When Faith is Tested*, author Jeffrey Zurheide[2] gives five possibilities: the deterministic answer (It is God's will)[3]; the didactic answer (God is teaching me something)[4]; the athletic answer (God is training me for something)[5]; God is a divine disciplinarian (God is punishing me)[6]. Zurheide comes out at a different place by working with this triad: God is good; God is great; evil is real. He uses all three of these components and posits: "theodicy is a mystery; suffering is at its core mystery; God is mystery."[7]

Earlier in this book, I talked about the death of our son, David, at age twenty-six with a child on the way. Why did God not answer my years of prayer for his safety? Why did God not allow him to recover from the accident?

I have shared my experience of healing in the confidence that you know that my prayers have not always been answered. I know that bargaining is not part of the process, but I would have taken the cancer if my son could have lived. I know that it does not work that way.

I do know that healing and curing come in many forms and faces. I do not have an answer to the lack of healing and curing as raised by the issue of theodicy. I will keep open to multivalent ways of healing and curing. As a theologian, maybe the point of theological inquiry is not to get closer to the answer, but to the mystery of God.

NOTES

1   Bidwell, Duane R., After the Worst Day Ever: What Sick Kids Know About Sustaining Hope in Chronic Illness (Boston: Beacon Press, 2024), p.3.
2   Jeffry R. Zurheide, *When Faith is Tested: Pastoral Responses to Suffering and Tragic Death* (Minneapolis: Fortress, 1977).
3   Zurheide, *When Faith is Tested*, 20.
4   Zurheide, *When Faith is Tested*, 21.
5   Zurheide, *When Faith is Tested*, 22,
6   Zurheide, *When Faith is Tested*, 23.
7   Zurheide, *When Faith is Tested*, 73.

Bibliography

CHAPTER 1

Abbey, Aoife. *Seven Signs of Life: Unforgettable Stories from an Intensive Care Doctor.* New York: Arcade Publishing, 2019.

Bearison, David J. *When Treatment Fails: How Medicine Cares for Dying Children.* New York: Oxford University Press, 2006.

Benson, Herbert and Marg Stark. *Timeless Healing: The Power of Biology and Belief.* New York: Simon and Schuster, 1996.

Bons-Storm, Riet. *The Incredible Woman: Listening to Women's Silences in Pastoral Care and Counseling.* Nashville: Abingdon Press, 1996.

Byrd, Randolph C. "Positive Therapeutic Effects of Intercessory Prayer in a Coronary Care Unit Population." Southern Medical Journal, 81, no. 7 (1998): 826–29. Doi: 10.1097/00007611-198807000-00005.

Chrysostom, John. "Homily III." Page 62 in *Homilies on the Gospel of St. Matthew (I-XLV).* Edited by Paul A. Boer Sr. Scotts Valley, CA: CreateSpace Publishing, 2012.

Cleaveland, Clif. *Sacred Space: Stories from a Life in Medicine.* Philadelphia: American College of Physicians, 1998.

Dunn, Mary. *Where Paralytics Walk and the Blind See: Stories of Sickness at the Juncture of Worlds.* Princeton: Princeton University Press, 2022.

Gawande, Atul. 2014. *Being Mortal: Medicine and What Matters in the End*. New York: Holt, 2014.

Hewitt Suchocki, Marjorie. *In God's Presence: Theological Reflections on Prayer*. Atlanta: Chalice, 1996.

Kelsey, Morton. *Healing and Christianity: A Classic Study*. Minneapolis: Augsburg, 1995.

Lusignan Schultz, Nancy. *Mrs. Mattingly's Miracle: The Prince, the Widow, and the Cure That Shocked the City*. New Haven: Yale University Press, 2011.

Matthews, Dale. 1996. "Plenary Address for the Spirituality and Healing in Medicine Conference." Boston, MA. Harvard Medical School, Deaconess Hospital, December 15–17, 1996.

Matthews, William. *A Collection of Affidavits and Certificates, Relative to the Wonderful Cure of Ann Mattingly, Which Took Place in the City of Washington, D.C., on the Tenth of March, 1824*. Washington, DC: Georgetown University Library, Special Collections, 1824.

Mohrmann, Margaret E. *Medicine as Ministry: Reflections on Suffering, Ethics, and Hope*. Cleveland: Pilgrim Press, 1995.

Morton, Nelle. *The Journey is Home*. Boston: Beacon, 1985.

Shimer, Porter. *Healing Secrets of the Native Americans: Herbs, Remedies, and Practices that Restore the Body, Mind, and Spirit*. New York: Tess Press, 1999.

CHAPTER 2

Barry, Jennifer. *Bishops in Flight: Exile and Displacement in Late Antiquity*. Oakland, CA: University of California Press, 2019.

Clark, Elizabeth A. "John Chrysostom and the 'Subintroductae.'" *Church History* 46, no.2 (1977): 171–85.

Duran, Eduardo. *Healing the Soul Wound*. New York: Teachers College Press, 2019.

Dykstra, Robert. *Images of Pastoral Care: Classic Readings.* Danvers, MA: Chalice Press, 2005.

Felitti, V. et al. "Relationship of Childhood Abuse and Household Dysfunction to Many of the Leading Causes of Death in Adults: The Adverse Childhood Experiences (ACE) Study." *American Journal of Preventive Medicine* 14, no.4 (1998): 245–58.

Guralnik, Orna. "I'm a Couples Therapist. Something New is Happening in Relationships." *The New York Times Magazine.* May 16, 2023. https://tinyurl.com/yk4eupmm.

Hartney, Aideen. *John Chrysostom and the Transformation of the City.* London: Duckworth, 2004.

Hilsman, Gordon J. "The Unconsciously Hidden: Potential Drinking Problems in the General Hospital." Pages 29 to 43 in *Confrontation in Spiritual Care: An Anthology for Clinical Caregivers.* Edited by Gordon J. Hilsman and Sandra Walker. Olympia: Summit Bay Press, 2022.

Holper, J. Frederick. "What does it mean to be ordained?" Presbyterianmission.org, 2022. https://tinyurl.com/2b9xf596.

Johnson Edwards, Lindsey. "Medicine and the Market: The Misenchantment of Modernity." Unpublished paper, Southern Methodist University, 2023.

Sion Mokhtarian, Jason. *Medicine in the Talmud: Natural and Supernatural Therapies between Magic and Science.* Oakland: University of California Press. 2022.

Spence, Joanne. *Trauma-Informed Yoga: A Toolbox for Therapists.* Eau Claire, WI: PESI Publishing, 2021.

Stevenson-Moessner, Jeanne. "The Impaired Healer." Unpublished paper, Southern Methodist University, 2023.

Van Der Kolk, Bessel. *The Body Keeps Scored: Brain, Mind, and Body in the Healing of Trauma.* New York: Penguin Books, 2014.

Wilson Van Veller, Courtney. "Paul's Therapy of the Soul: A New Approach to John Chrysostom and Anti-Judaism." PhD diss., Boston University, 2015.

CHAPTER 3

Bauer, Walter, and William Arndt, Wilbur F. Gingrich. *A Greek-English Lexicon of the New Testament and Other Early Christian Literature.* Chicago: University of Chicago Press, 2001.

Bynum, William. *The History of Medicine: A Very Short Introduction.* New York: Oxford University Press, 2008.

Cleaveland, Clif. *Sacred Space: Stories from a Life in Medicine.* Philadelphia: American College of Physicians, 1998.

Duran, Eduardo. *Healing the Soul Wound: Trauma Informed Counseling for Indigenous Communities,* 2nd ed. New York: Teachers College Press of Columbia University, 2019.

Edelstein, Ludwig. *From The Hippocratic Oath: Text, Translation, and Interpretation.* Baltimore: Johns Hopkins Press, 1943.

Fortune, Marie. *Is Nothing Sacred? When Sex Invades the Pastoral Relationship.* San Francisco: Harper, 1992.

Gambee Henry, Linda and James Douglas Henry. *Reclaiming Soul in Health Care: Practical Strategies for Revitalizing Providers of Care.* Chicago: American Hospital Association Press, 1999.

Graham, Ruth. "Sex Abuse in Catholic Church: Over 1,900 Minors Abused in Illinois, State Says." *The New York Times.* May 23, 2023. https://www.nytimes.com/2023/05/23/us/illinois-catholic-church-sex-abuse.html?unlocked_article_code=1.CU0.hGKI.BnkuoRGkc-ew&smid=url-share.

Hagood, Susan Lee. "Witness to Christ, Witness to Pain: One Women's Journey Through Wife Battering." Pages 11–22 in *Sermons Seldom Heard: Women Proclaim Their Lives*. Edited by Annie Lally Milhaven. New York: Crossroad Press, 1991.

Hamilton, J. S. "Scribonius Largus on the Medical Profession," *Bull Hist Med* 60 (1986): 209–16.

Hayes, Evan and Stephen Nimis. *Hippocrates' On Airs, Waters and Places and the Hippocratic Oath: An Intermediate Greek Reader*. Oxford, OH: Faenum Publishing, 2013.

Horney, Karen. *Feminine Psychology*. New York: Norton, 1967.

Lord, G.E.R. Introduction to *Hippocratic Writings*. London: Penguin Books, 1978.

Miles, Stephen M. *The Hippocratic Oath and the Ethics of Medicine*. New York: Oxford University Press, 2004.

Pellegrino, Edmund. "Humanism and Ethics in Roman Medicine: Translation and Commentary on a Text of Scribonius Largus." *Lit Med* 7 (1988): 22–38.

Porter, Ray. *Medicine: A History of Healing*. New York: Barnes & Noble, 1997.

Skloot, Rebecca. *The Immortal Life of Henrietta Lacks*. New York: Random House, 2010.

Stark, Rodney. *The Rise of Christianity*. Princeton: Princeton University Press, 1996.

Stevenson-Moessner, Jeanne. Preface in *Women Out of Order: Risking Change and Creating Care in a Multicultural World*. Edited by Jeanne Stevenson-Moessner and Bishop Teresa Snorton. Minneapolis: Fortress Press, 2000.

Sulmsy, Daniel P. *The Healer's Calling: A Spirituality for Physicians and Other Health Care Professionals*. New York: Paulist, 1997.

Sweet, Victoria. *God's Hotel: A Doctor, A Hospital, and a Pilgrimage to the Heart of Medicine*. New York: Riverhead, 2012.

CHAPTER 4

Dyson, Michael Eric. *Pride*. Oxford: Oxford University Press, 2006.

Erikson, Erik. *Childhood and Society*, 2nd ed. New York: Norton, 1993.

Fairlie, Henry. *The Seven Deadly Sins Today*. Washington: New Republic Books, 1978.

Kee, H. C. "Testaments of the Twelve Patriarchs (Second Century BCE)." Pages 782–83 in *The Old Testament Pseudepigrapha: Apocalyptic Literature and Testaments*. Edited by James Charlesworth. Garden City: Doubleday, 2008.

Kleinberg, Aviad. *Seven Deadly Sins: A Very Partial List*. Cambridge: Harvard University Press, 2008.

Konydyk DeYoung, Rebecca. "The Seven Deadly Sins." Page 25 in vol. 5 (Si-Z) *The Encyclopedia of Christianity*. Grand Rapids: Eerdmans, 2008.

Mayer, Wendy. "John Chrysostom: Moral Philosopher and Physician of the Soul." Pages 193–216 in *John Chrysostom: Past, Present, and Future*. Edited by Doru Costache and Mario Baghos. Sydney: AICOS Press, 2017.

McDougal, Joy Ann. "Sin—No More? A Feminist Re-Visioning of a Christian Theology of Sin." *Anglican Theological Review* 88 (2006): 215–35.

Miller, Jean Baker. *Toward a New Psychology of Women*. Boston: Beacon Press, 1976.

Redmond, Sheila A. "Christian 'Virtues' and Recovery from Child Sexual Abuse." Pages 70–88 in *Christianity, Patriarchy, and Abuse: A Feminist Critique*. Edited by Joanne Carlson Brown and Carole R. Bohn. New York: Pilgrim Press, 1989.

Saiving Goldstein, Valerie. "The Human Situation: A Feminine View," *Journal of Religion* 40, no. 100 (1960): 100–12.

Stevenson-Moessner, Jeanne. "A New Pastoral Paradigm and Practice." Pages 200–4 in *Women in Travail and Transition: A New Pastoral Care*. Edited by Maxine Glaz and Jeanne Stevenson-Moessner. Minneapolis: Fortress Press, 1991.

———. *In Her Own Time: Women and Developmental Issues in Pastoral Theology*. Minneapolis: Fortress Press, 2000.

———. *Prelude to Practical Theology: Variations on Theory and Practice*. Nashville: Abingdon, 2008.

CHAPTER 5

Buc, Hannah Loring Murphy. *Ain't Never Been Cared For: A Grounded Theory of Receiving Hospice and Palliative Care for Homeless and Vulnerably Houses Individuals*. Unpublished PhD diss., Catholic University of America, 2023.

Cadge, Wendy. *Spiritual Care: The Everyday Work of Chaplains*. Oxford: Oxford University Press, 2022.

Cleary, James. "The Robin Hood of Opioids: Palliative Care in the Underdeveloped World." Pages 155–63 in *The Pursuit of Life: The Promise and Challenge of Palliative Care*. Edited by Robert Fine and Jack Levison. University Park, PA: Pennsylvania State University Press, 2023.

Craddock, Fred. *The Spirit of Adoption: At Home in God's Family*. Louisville: Westminster John Knox, 2003.

Duran, Eduardo. *Healing the Soul Wound: Trauma-Informed Counseling for Indigenous Communities*, 2nd ed. New York: Teachers College Press, 2019.

Fine, Robert, and Jack Levison. *The Pursuit of Life: The Promise and Challenge of Palliative Care*. Edited by Robert Fine and Jack Levison. University Park, PA: Pennsylvania State University Press, 2023.

Frankl, Viktor E. *The Doctor and the Soul: From Psychotherapy to Logotherapy,* 3rd ed. New York: Penguin Press, 1955.

Gafney, Wil. "Gonna Take a Miracle." *Womanists Wading in the Word.* https://www.wilgafney.com/2023/02/05/gonna-take-a-miracle/.

Grant, Paul Glen. *Healing and Power in Ghana: Early Indigenous Expressions of Christianity.* Waco: Baylor University Press, 2020.

Hordern, Joshua. *Compassion in Healthcare: Pilgrimage, Practice, and Civil Life.* Oxford: Oxford University Press, 2020.

Mayer, Wendy. "Shaping the Sick Soul: Reshaping the Identity of John Chrysostom." Pages 140–64 in *Christians Shaping Identity from the Roman Empire to Byzantium: Inspired by Pauline Allen.* Supplements to Vigilae Christianae 132. Leiden: Brill, 2015.

Pollan, Michal. *How to Change Your Mind: What the New Science of Psychedelics Teaches Us About Consciousness, Dying, Addiction, Depression, and Transcendence.* New York: Penguin Press, 2018.

Roberts, Matthias. "How I Find Healing from Religious Trauma." *Sojourners Magazine,* 2023, pages 23–27. ISSN 0364-2097. https://sojo.net/magazine/septemberoctober-2023/healing-from-religious-trauma.

Scott, Buddy. "Arms of Christ Mural Embraces Medical Profession History," *The Facts: Covering Brazoria County,* 2011. https://tinyurl.com/ykb7ea2n.

Slade, Darren M. "Adverse Religious Experiences (AREs) vs. Religious Trauma (RT): An Important Distinction," *Global Center for Religious Research Academic Institute,* 2022. https://www.gcrr.org/post/adversereligiousexperiences.

Suchocki, Marjorie Hewitt. *In God's Presence: Theological Reflections on Prayer.* St. Louis: Chalice Press, 1996.

Thomas, Debbie. "Why and How I Believe in Miracles," *The Christian Century*, 2023. https://www.christiancentury.org/believing-in-miracles.

Whang, Oliver. "A Rural Doctor Gave Her All. Then Her Heart Broke," *New York Times*, 2022. https://tinyurl.com/2wmsanze.

EPILOGUE

Zurheide, Jeffry R. *When Faith is Tested: Pastoral Responses to Suffering and Tragic Death*. Minneapolis: Fortress Press, 1977.

Index